CANCER
AND
GENETICS

ANSWERING YOUR PATIENTS' QUESTIONS

A Manual for Clinicians and Their Patients

From the American Cancer Society and PRR, Inc.

Written by
Randi Londer Gould

In consultation with
Henry T. Lynch, MD
Creighton University School of Medicine

Robert A. Smith, PhD
American Cancer Society

James F. McCarthy
PRR, Inc.

Illustrations by Jeanne Kelly
Aardvark Design

Clinical opinions expressed in this book are those of the authorities quoted and do not necessarily reflect the opinions of the sponsors, writers, editors, or the publisher and officers of PRR, Inc., or of the American Cancer Society.

Copyright ©1997 by PRR, Inc., and the American Cancer Society. All rights reserved. This book is protected by copyright. No part of it may be reproduced in any manner or by any means, electronic or mechanical, without the written permission of the publisher.

Library of Congress Catalog Card Number 97-065337.

ISBN 9641823-6-x

Single copies of this book are available at $15.95 each. For information on bulk quantities, contact the publishers, PRR, Inc., 17 Prospect Street, Huntington, NY 11743. Telephone: (516) 424-8900.

Printed in the U.S.A.

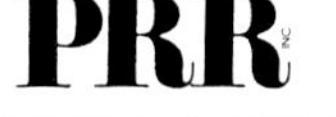

Publishers of ONCOLOGY
Oncology News International
Cancer Management
Primary Care & Cancer
Medical Oncology:
A Comprehensive Review
Cancer Management:
A Multidisciplinary Approach

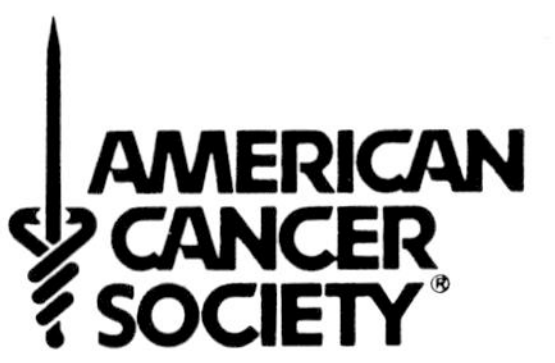

To Martin D. Gould
and
Rowena and Sam Levine

Taken too soon

RLG

Acknowledgements

This manual on the genetics of cancer is a joint venture of PRR, Inc. and the American Cancer Society. PRR is the publisher of ONCOLOGY, Oncology News International, Primary Care & Cancer, Cancer Management, and various textbooks and treatment manuals. The content of the manual is based in part on the proceedings of an American Cancer Society conference: Workshop On Heritable Cancer Syndromes and Genetic Testing. The book contains generous portions of expertise from speakers at that workshop, but especially from the following:

Judy Garber, MD
*Assistant Professor
of Medicine
Department of Cancer
Epidemiology and Control
Dana-Farber Cancer Institute
Harvard Medical School*

Stephen J. Lemon, MD
*Assistant Professor
Department of
Preventive Medicine
Creighton University
School of Medicine*

Henry T. Lynch, MD
*Chairman, Department
of Preventive Medicine
Creighton University
School of Medicine*

Robert A. Smith, PhD
*Senior Director
Cancer Detection
and Treatment
American Cancer Society*

Kenneth Offit, MD
*Chief, Clinical Genetics
Service Research
Memorial Sloan-Kettering
Cancer Center*

June Peters, MS
*Genetics Counselor
Medical Genetics Branch
National Center for Human
Genome Research
National Institutes
of Health*

Karen Rothenberg, JD, MPA
*Marjorie Cook
Professor of Law
University of Maryland
School of Law*

Susan Tinley, MS
*Genetics Counselor
Department of
Preventive Medicine
Creighton University
School of Medicine*

Contents

INTRODUCTION

A Complicated Question

Henry T. Greely, JD
Professor of Law and Professor, by courtesy, of Genetics
Stanford Universty

Retinoblastoma, Li-Fraumeni Syndrome, Fanconi's anemia, hereditary medullary thyroid cancer. Breast cancer, ovarian cancer, prostate cancer, colon cancer. The articles keep on coming, linking more cancers—and more common cancers—to inherited genes. Doctors see them in medical journals, patients see them in newspapers and magazines, and both wonder what they mean. Research is outrunning the understanding of both physicians and patients.

This book is an effort to even the balance, at least in part. The American Cancer Society, with PRR, Inc., has tried to lay out basic information about the inheritance of cancer risks in ways that can help both medical professionals and interested patients begin to grasp the issues. As co-chair of a Stanford Working Group on Genetic Testing for Breast Cancer Susceptibility, I too grappled with these questions. I have concluded that, in looking at genetic testing for cancer risk, physicians and patients need to keep in mind two important general principles: every test is different - and every test is the same.

Whether genetic testing makes sense for any given patient will always be a complicated question. From the patient's perspective, a positive test result may lead to some useful medical interventions and to an increased ability to plan for the future, but it might also lead to increased personal anxiety, familial tensions, and employment or insurance discrimination. A negative test result would usually lead to some relief from anxiety, some increased ability to plan for the future, and perhaps some change in an existing regimen of cancer prevention or detection. For any individual patient, whether those likely outcomes make testing worthwhile will depend on many factors.

Complex Differences

Some of those factors will revolve around the genetics of this inherited risk. How is this increased risk inherited—is the trait dominant, recessive, X-linked, or something else? Does the patient's family history indicate that the patient really may be at increased genetic risk? How strong is the link between the genetic risk and the likelihood of cancer, both in terms of relative risk and absolute risk? A test result that shows a patient at a relative risk 10 times higher than that of the general population may mean one thing if the absolute risk has gone from 0.1% to 1% and quite another if it has gone from 5% to 50%.

Some of the factors will be medical. What is the cancer involved? At what age does it typically occur? How serious is the disease? Are there useful preventive measures that can be taken? Are there good treatments? Patients would appropriately have different views of heightened risks of ovarian cancer, prostate cancer, and squamous cell skin cancer.

Some of the factors will relate to the test itself. At what stage in life is it being offered—before conception, prenatally, to a child, or to an adult? How accurate is it, in terms of both false positives and false negatives? Does it require that affected family members provide DNA samples? How expensive is it and will insurance cover it?

The most important factors are likely to be personal. What psychological effects would the test results, positive or negative, be likely to have on this patient? What is the patient's family structure and how would those family members— spouses, parents, siblings, children, and others—react to the test results? Could this patient face loss of health insurance, life insurance, or employment as a result of the test results? What is the patient's reaction to cancer in general? What is the patient's personal experience with the disease? How much knowledge does this individual patient want?

In a very real sense, the issue of genetic testing for cancer susceptibility will be different for every cancer, for every test, and for every patient. And, to make things even more complicated, almost all of the factors mentioned above are in flux, as new genetic research, new cancer treatments, and new legislation change the status quo.

The Important Similarities

If every test is different, what good can come from a relatively short manual? All tests are different, but, in other respects, all the tests are the same. It is in highlighting these similarities that this manual can be particularly valuable.

For all of these tests, informed consent is likely to be particularly important. There will not often be obvious medical answers about the value of the tests; the dominant considerations are likely to be personal. Only the patient can assess those considerations and patients can only make good decisions if they have good information.

The process of informed consent needs to alert patients to the importance of the non-medical issues. Patients may need to be told to think about the effects of test results, positive or negative, on their family, on their own psychological well-being, and on their health insurance or job.

Patients will need access to follow-up care. Those who test positive will need to talk about the medical implications; they may need psychological help. Those who test negative may also need counseling with their test results. It would be tragic if women who tested negative for an increased genetic risk of breast cancer decided to dispense forever with breast examinations and mammography.

Professionals advising these patients must know what they are talking about and the information they will need to convey —genetic, medical, and personal—is too important, too complex, too new, and too rapidly changing for competence to be assumed. Competence will not be the province of any one profession or specialty, but neither can it be assumed that genetic counselors, primary care physicians, oncologists, or anyone else will *necessarily* know enough about the genetic testing for cancer risk to do more good than harm.

This manual is one useful step toward creating such competence. It is not the final word, but it gives both professionals and concerned patients a place to start. Its value lies in both the substantive information it conveys and in the leads it gives for further information, from the literature and from experts in the field. The annual update of this guide for clinicians will be particularly important in such a rapidly evolving field.

We live in exciting times and research into the genetics of cancer are one part of that excitement. We all share an obligation to ensure that this research is used in ways that improve lives, not harm them.

—Henry T. Greely, JD

Cancer and Genetics: The Primary Care Physician's Role in Counseling and Testing

Henry T. Lynch, MD
Professor and Chairman, Department of Preventive
Medicine and Public Health and Professor of Medicine
and Director, Creighton Cancer Center, Creighton
University, Omaha, Nebraska

With the explosive progress that has been made in cancer genetics in general and molecular genetics in particular over the past decade, we seem to read and hear about some new discovery regarding "cancer genes" almost daily in our local newspapers and television news programs. For example, the discovery of "cancer-prone genes" and the identification of "new" hereditary cancer syndromes have had extensive coverage in both the scientific and lay press. As a result, patients around the world have been avidly seeking information from their physicians about how genes may be controlling their cancer destiny. Thus, we have prepared this manual in order to help you explain this complex subject to your patients in easy to understand language. We have also provided analogies and illustrations that most patients will easily comprehend.

In many instances, you may well want to give the manual to patients to read certain sections. For that very reason, we have kept the language in the booklet at a level they will understand. Thus, with your own deeper knowledge and understanding of genetics, plus this basic explanation, you will have a very usable guide to explain the genetics of cancer.

For some patients, the slightest evidence of cancer in their family may provoke crippling fright and anxiety. In some individuals, such responses may partially be due to their misinterpretation of the media accounts. Occasionally, however, the media presentations may be wholly or substantially inaccurate. The reports may have played down the importance of genetics in a particular cancer, giving patients a false sense of security or, alternatively, may have exaggerated genetic risk factors, thereby provoking unnecessary alarm and instigating expensive cancer screening.

A subset of these concerned patients may request some form of immediate remedial action, such as prophylactic removal of their breasts or ovaries, even though there may not be any solid genetic basis for their perception of increased cancer risk. In each case, it becomes the physician's responsibility to accurately interpret whether there is a reality base for patients' concerns about their genetic risk and to counsel them accordingly.

The Physician's Responsibilities

This requires that the physician accrue a sufficiently detailed family history with adequate documentation of cancer occurrences at all anatomic sites in order to formulate (or rule out) a hereditary cancer syndrome diagnosis. If such a diagnosis is established, the patient then needs to be informed about his or her personal risk for cancer and about available surveillance and management strategies, including their advantages and limitations. Again, this manual is aimed at helping you reassure and advise your patients.

When DNA testing is indicated, an explanation of the testing procedure must be conveyed to the patient. The possible penalties of genetic disclosure must be discussed as well. For example, there is a risk that insurance companies may refuse coverage for cancer surveillance or even surgical prophylaxis (such as prophylactic oophorectomy in a BRCA1 carrier) because it is a "preexisting condition" or designate gene carriers as "uninsurable." Employers, especially those with self-insurance, may find it in their financial interest to discriminate against gene carriers.

As with any family, families with hereditary cancer are composed of individuals, with different emotional traits, experiences, and motivations that influence personal decisions. The results of gene testing for one individual may reveal the gene status of another who is adamantly opposed to that revelation. The emotional impact of identification as a gene carrier will vary from one individual to another, but patients need to be encouraged to anticipate their own reaction based on past experiences and existing support systems. Even noncarriers may feel guilty about their gene status (so-called survivor guilt). Clearly, all of these matters are integral features of the genetic counseling process.

Chapter 7 will help you avoid some of the sand traps in the family aspects of genetic counseling and testing for cancer.

Four Important Questions

Are physicians sufficiently knowledgeable and ready to perform genetic counseling? Are they adequately trained to supervise cancer genetic counselors? Are guidelines for cancer genetic counseling available? Are there enough available certified genetic counselors who are sufficiently knowledgeable about cancer genetics and the natural history of these disorders? This knowledge is essential so that patients can receive, and intelligently act upon, recommendations based on accurate genetic risk information, so that, in turn, appropriate choices about surveillance and management strategies (inclusive of their limitations) can be entertained. Again, this manual will help answer these questions for you and your patients.

A gap exists between what is known about cancer genetics and patients' counseling needs and their demands for information and realistic cancer prevention measures. Such a state of affairs should not be surprising, however, given the embryonic status of the newly emerging disciplines of cancer genetics and molecular genetics. For example, we are still low on the learning curve relative to our understanding of the variation in penetrance and expression of cancer-prone genes, particularly with respect to age of onset, tumor spectrum, pathology, and prognosis. Questions about each of these issues abound.

We also have insufficient information about the multifaceted legal, ethical, and moral issues that may impact on genetic counseling. For example, what is the potential for malpractice litigation that may emanate from the genetic counseling process?

Appropriate Action Needed

The list of potential concerns about genetic counseling in hereditary cancer could be extended almost interminably. While full and complete answers to these questions may require many years of research (and some may be so elusive as to never be fully clarified), we, nevertheless, must appreciate the fact that if the medical community does not take appropriate action about cancer genetic diagnosis, genetic counseling, and management, patients will seek advice from individuals with less training. Given market demands, untrained health-care professionals may be pressured into providing services with implications that they neither understand nor appreciate.

Given that trained cancer genetics counselors are not available in every community, and that the primary care physician is usually the first person a patient seeks out with medical questions, it behooves family physicians, general internists, and gynecologists to familiarize themselves with the basics of genetic testing/counseling for cancer. This manual is meant to supplement your own knowledge of the subject and help you better address your patients' concerns.

—Henry T. Lynch, MD

Physicians in primary care may choose to incorporate hereditary breast or ovarian cancer risk assessment in the initial patient consultation. A patient who has a strong family history of breast or ovarian cancer may be an appropriate candidate for BRCA1 and BRCA2 genetic susceptibility testing.

BRACAnalysis™ Checklist for Physicians

Myriad Genetic Laboratories recommends that physicians follow these steps when considering or referring patients for BRACAnalysis™:

☐ **1.** Obtain a detailed medical and family history to ensure the patient is an appropriate candidate for BRACAnalysis™.

☐ **2.** If the patient is a candidate for testing, recommend pretest and post-test education and genetic counseling by a qualified health care professional.

☐ **3.** For patients who elect to be tested, review informed consent with the patient and obtain patient's signature.

☐ **4.** Complete the BRACAnalysis™ Test Request Form, supplied in Myriad's *Specimen Collection & Transportation Kit.*

☐ **5.** Obtain a blood sample.

---

*To order **BRACAnalysis**™ physician and patient educational resources, or to speak with a health care professional about genetic susceptibility testing for your patients, call Myriad Client Services at (800) 469-7423.*

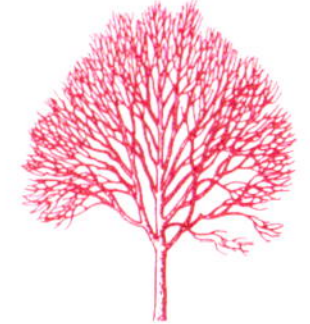

Myriad Genetic Laboratories

320 Wakara Way ■ Salt Lake City, Utah 84108

For more information: Toll free (800) 469-7423 ■ FAX (801) 584-3615
e-mail BRACA@myriad.com ■ website http://www.myriad.com

Tear out and retain for reference

Evaluating Your Patient's Risk for Hereditary Breast and Ovarian Cancer

1. DOES THE PATIENT HAVE A FIRST-DEGREE BLOOD RELATIVE (MALE OR FEMALE) WITH A KNOWN BRCA1 OR BRCA2 MUTATION?

☐ *Yes* ☐ *No*

2. HAS THE PATIENT EVER BEEN DIAGNOSED WITH CANCER? IF SO, HOW OLD WAS SHE AT DIAGNOSIS?

	YES/NO	AGE AT DIAGNOSIS
Breast Cancer		
Ovarian Cancer		
Other cancer(s)		

3. DOES THE PATIENT BELONG TO AN ETHNIC GROUP (FOR INSTANCE, ASHKENAZI JEWISH) THAT HAS AN INCREASED INCIDENCE OF INHERITED MUTATIONS IN BRCA1 OR BRCA2?

☐ *Yes* ☐ *No*

4. DOES THE PATIENT HAVE RELATIVES WHO HAVE BEEN DIAGNOSED WITH BREAST CANCER OR OVARIAN CANCER?

RELATIVE	BREAST	OVARIAN	AGE AT DIAGNOSIS
Mother			
Sister			
Daughter			
Grandmother			
Aunt			
Cousin			
Other (specify)			

Special Considerations:
- *Ensure you have considered both maternal and paternal sides of the family.*
- *Ask clarifying questions to help the patient distinguish between when a cancer was diagnosed (age of onset) and when a relative may have died of the disease.*
- *Follow up on vaguely suggestive findings, such as a history of "female cancers" in one or more blood relatives.*

Note: This form has been adapted from the Pretest Checklist for Physicians, available from Myriad Genetic Laboratories.

CHAPTER I

The Age of Genetics Is Upon Us

"Genetic technology is hurtling down the track."

—*Francis S. Collins, MD, PhD*
Director, National Center
for Human Genome Research

What can you tell patients who come to your office waving the latest press report heralding this week's finding on genetics and cancer? Researchers mapping the human genome have made grand predictions: With a "Complete Travel Guide To Our Genes" they say, eventually we will test for and treat—perhaps even prevent—any of the more than 4,000 genetic diseases.

The "gene-ie" has slipped out of the bottle. And it's not going back in.

Already, scientists have unearthed the chromosomes' genetic loci of more than a dozen cancers. With the advent of PCR—polymerase chain reaction, a sort of super-Xerox for DNA—the pace of cloning and characterizing genes shot ahead. Now sequencing technology, which helps fill in the blanks on genetic maps, will soon crank up much faster and cheaper. Scientists at the University of Michigan have built a credit-card-sized sequencer. This silicon chip threatens to generate an avalanche of genetic information. By the year 2005 or even sooner, researchers expect to map the entire human genome, finding all our 100,000 genes.

This research hikes patients' expectations—and anxiety. Where can I get tested for cancer susceptibility genes? What do I do if I have bad genes? Will presently available screening and management tools save my life? Can gene therapy cure my child's illness? As primary health care providers, you and your staff will find yourselves fielding such questions more and more. And it may disappoint some patients to learn that the giant strides of genetic science have outpaced our ability to make use of many of the findings.

It's important to bear in mind that relatively few cancers in the general population—maybe 5% to 10%—are inherited. While all types of cancer are genetic, in the sense that the disease stems from gene malfunction, most people who contract breast or colon cancer—even a small fraction of those in families with a history of these diseases—have not fallen heir to faulty genes. Somewhere along the way they acquired a genetic mutation: Exposure to a toxic chemical, or a blunder made during cell division tweaked their DNA. Such "sporadic" cancers occur so commonly they can cluster in families purely by chance, usually among the older generations.

Rating the Risks

Knowing where inherited cancer genes lurk on the chromosomes does answer some questions, but it also raises a raft of other issues that bear on whether patients should seek testing now. To explore those issues, the National Institutes of Health and the Department of Energy have formed a joint Task Force on Genetic Testing. Among the topics they are considering:

- Genetic tests can predict the risk of future disease, but they cannot gauge that risk with any great certainty. For instance, at least 15% of patients with a mutation on the BRCA1 breast-ovarian cancer gene do not develop the disease. A mutated gene's "penetrance," or likelihood of causing disease, determines this number. These people may be predisposed to cancer, but not ill-fated. And those who carry weaker susceptibility genes for other cancers can also escape disease. Another issue: Quite often, no independent test can confirm predictions; proof comes only when the disease appears.
- Medical science cannot always point toward the best path of treatment options. We may have grasped a disease gene yesterday, but find ourselves still unable to manage it today. What should a healthy patient do if she knows she is at risk for disease? Increase her cancer screening? Opt for prophylactic surgery? Watch and wait?
- Genetic information can put patients at risk of stigma and even discrimination. A recent study published in *Science* found that

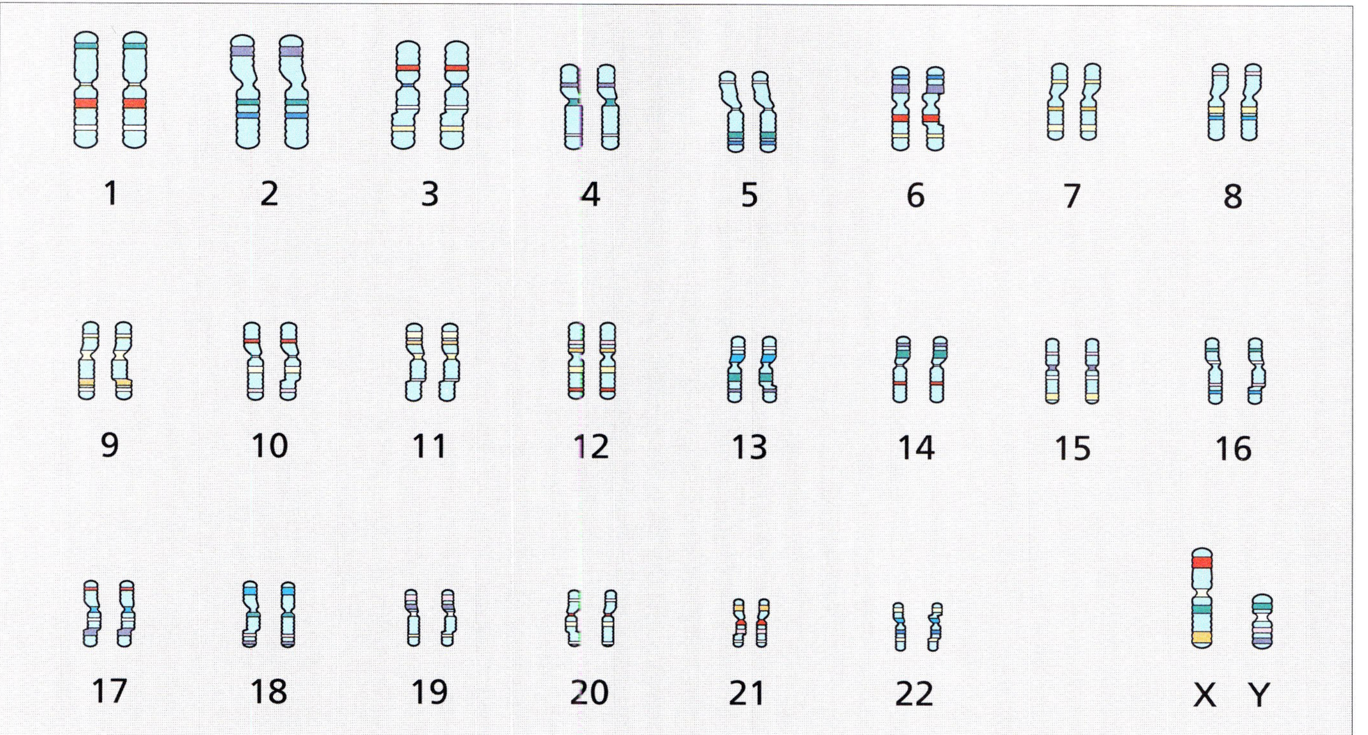

Figure 1: The human male karyotype—the chromosomes wherein the genes reside. Each person's karyotype is different.

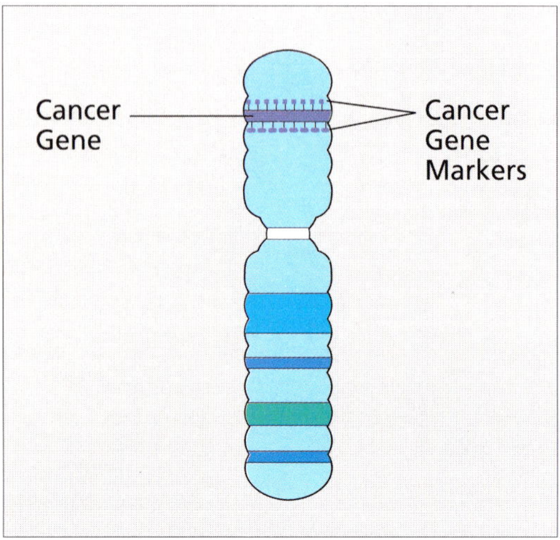

Figure 2: In narrowing the search for a specific gene, researchers often identify gene markers—characteristic segments of DNA or genes for known traits—that lie close to the target gene and are inherited along with it.

nearly half of people asked on health insurance applications about a family history of genetic diseases were later turned down for coverage. Most subjects in the study said they would not want their insurers to know they were tested. Some respondents believed they were denied a job or fired because of a genetic disorder. Currently, no federal laws exist that would protect this information from the prying eyes of insurance companies or from present and future employers.

Much magical thinking surrounds the notion of "bad genes." Some people believe they are somehow responsible for passing on mutations to their children; others may feel "unfit" for possessing a faulty gene. Conversely, when one member of a cancer-prone family dodges the genetic bullet, he or she may feel guilty. Genetic findings can strain even the strongest of family bonds with feelings of shame, blame, guilt and anger bubbling up.

• Fewer than 2,000 trained genetic counselors work in the United States now. Most help prospective parents with prenatal tests for such conditions as Down's syndrome, spina bifida, and Tay-Sachs. Fewer than 200 specialize in genetics and cancer. Overburdened, they cannot possibly cope with the coming onslaught of patient demand.

The Shape of Things to Come

At this point, says Francis Collins, MD, genetic testing technology "may be more of a thorn in our sides than an advantage, but here it is and it's not going to go away." Dr.

Collins, who heads the Human Genome Research Project, worries that the technology may "prematurely find its way into clinical practice before we really know what it's worth."

In fact, the technology train has already left the station. It's bearing down now on patients in the form of direct marketing. Advertisements have targeted ethnic groups with higher cancer risk. Offering to screen Ashkenazi Jewish women for the breast cancer genes BRCA1 and BRCA2 at a cost of around $2,000, biotech companies hope to jump up demand for their services. Their ads promise results in 2 weeks on blood samples sent in by physicians. These companies provide counseling over the phone. That's far less than ideal when what they reveal may overwhelm, confuse or frighten patients.

Few government regulations on testing protect such patients. And the commercial screening companies have already leapfrogged over doctors and scientists who are just now hammering out recommendations on such issues as informed consent and other standards.

The National Cancer Genetics Network

To help physicians swing through the learning curve of molecular medicine, the National Cancer Institute aims to set up the National Cancer Genetics Network. The network will create a series of centers to focus on cancer genetics education, enrolling patients in standardized research protocols, risk assessment, testing and counseling. By amassing patient registries at these centers, follow-up intervention trials can zero in on individuals at high risk, not easy to pinpoint at present. The centers will use as their model the Cooperative Groups which have successfully profiled the risks and benefits of chemotherapy.

But because the wheels of bureaucracy creak slowly, these centers may not begin to operate until the end of 1997. Meanwhile, market forces will keep gliding along their much more well-oiled track as commercial concerns try to hold sway over potential breast and ovarian cancer patients.

The American Medical Association and American Nursing Association are also gearing up to help doctors, nurses, nurse practitioners, social workers, physician assistants and others to prepare for this new era of genetic testing. Called the National Coalition for Health Professional Education in Genetics, the program will provide educational materials and toughen up Board exams to reflect the need for this knowledge.

Knowing the Unknown

Family physicians have always had to deal with uncertainties when giving their patients new and emerging information. So why the urgency about cancer genetics? In many ways, this field differs qualitatively. Experts see it as:

- Personal. What could be more individual than one's DNA?
- Predictive. Unlike most medical tests, genetic tests give healthy people information about potential future risk, an eerie and possibly scary prospect. Not only can DNA tell us *where* cancer will occur (in the breast, ovary, or colon, for instance) but it can forecast approximately *when* the disease will strike—usually 15 to 20 years earlier than expected. It can even warn about the propensity for patients to develop other cancers in a syndrome.
- Powerful. The information has the power to change the course of lives, plans, behaviors.
- Private. It's still not certain how and from whom to shield genetic information. Who will have access to these records? Employers? Insurance carriers? Potential marital partners?
- Pedigree-sensitive. The information affects not just your patients but their relatives. What is your obligation to them?
- Permanent. Until gene therapy can make a lasting change in one's genome, the results are here to stay.
- Prejudicial. Even the whiff of potential disease could create discrimination or stigma.

How This Book Can Help

The challenge for those in the health profession is to navigate the winding path of genetic testing and molecular medicine, a path that sprouts new byways nearly every day. This book can help guide you down that road. Use it as a refresher course in genetics. Use it to help answer specific questions from patients concerned about cancer of the breast, ovary, colon, as well as the more rare inherited cancers. Consider sharing this book with your patients, keeping a copy in the waiting room. With this volume you will learn the step-by-step method for constructing a pedigree to better visualize the extent of cancer in a patient's family so that you can know when you need to refer a patient to a geneticist. In many cases, a patient's desire for genetic testing may arise from an exaggerated sense of risk; by using the information in this book you can provide perspective.

Also outlined: the genetic test, what it shows, and the laboratories qualified to conduct those tests. Counseling patients who seek genetic testing requires finely tuned listening skills. Through case histories we illustrate the many family issues that can arise when one member uncovers information that others might prefer to leave untouched. This volume also reports the most current state of legal affairs. As of now, legislators have yet to face squarely privacy issues. We discuss the implications for privacy, as well as discrimination on the job and in health insurance coverage.

The ancient Greek dramatist Sophocles warned that "it is but sorrow to be wise when wisdom profits not." While the promise of molecular genetics may be great, it is a promise not yet fulfilled. As the field evolves, we have to ensure that the technology does more good than harm. That will depend, in part, on primary care providers. Your patients will look to you to show them what they can expect from this newest revolution in medicine, and whether it can truly improve their lives now.

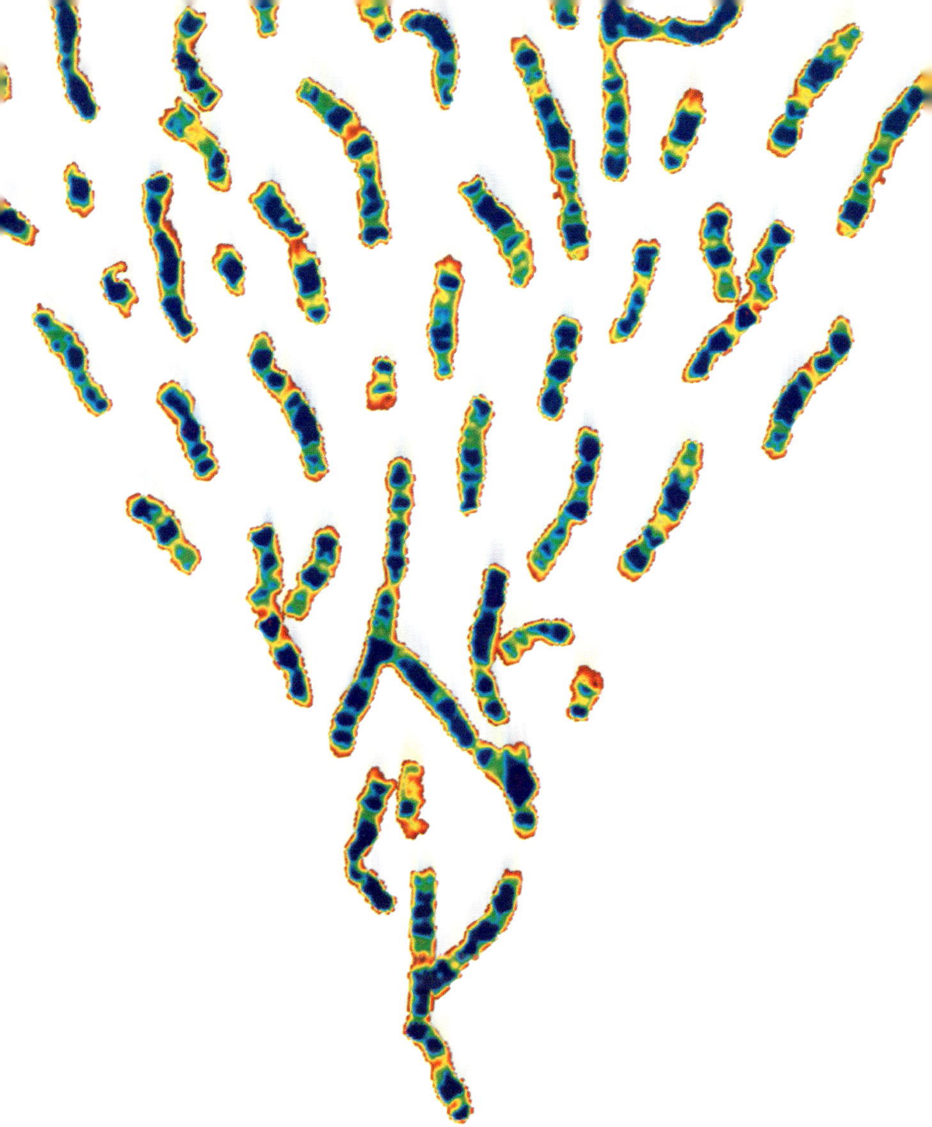

A new force in gene therapy

Creating a new and expanded vision in
gene therapy and cancer research.

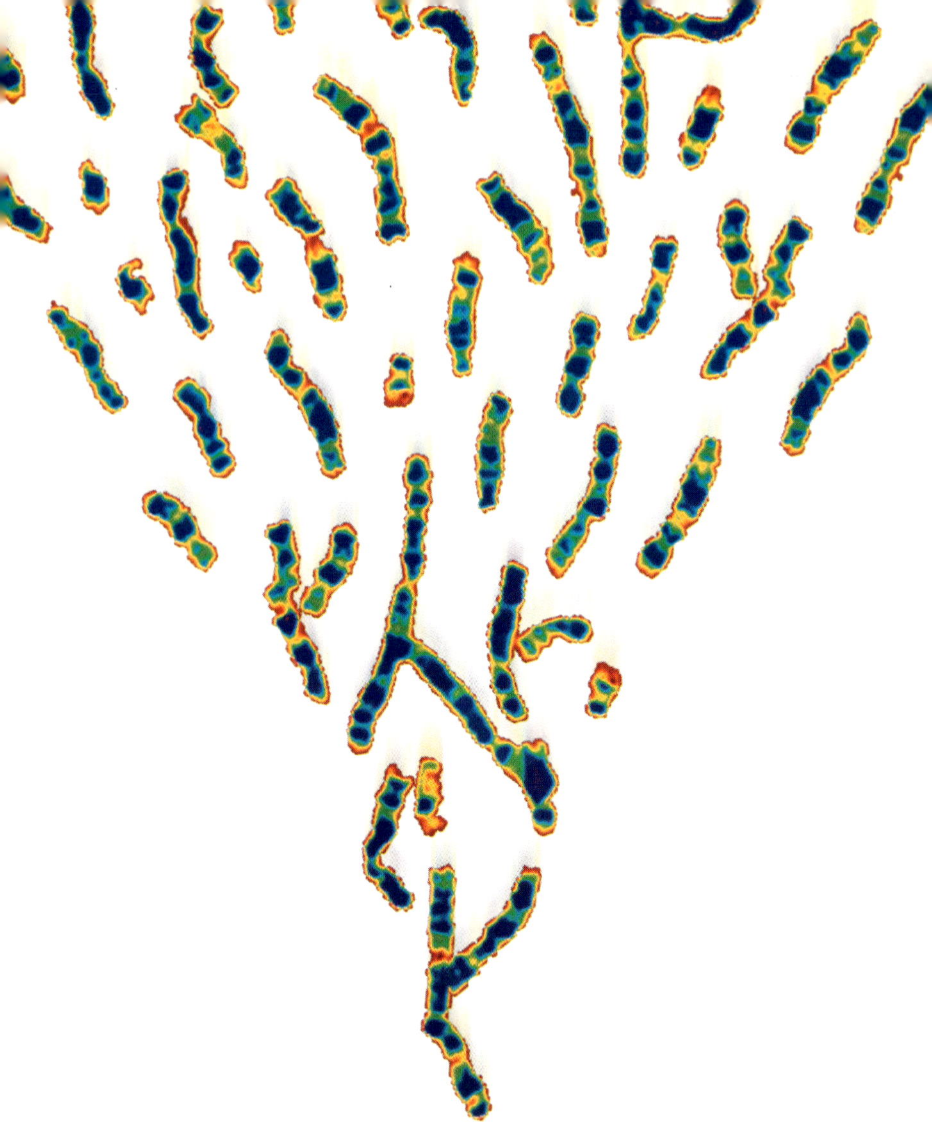

A new force in gene therapy

Creating a new and expanded vision in
gene therapy and cancer research.

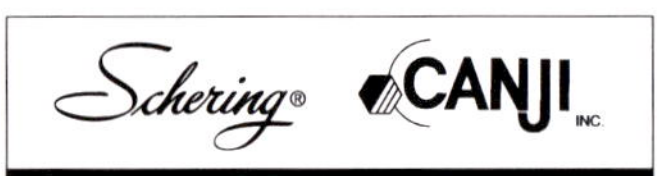

CHAPTER 2

Cancer Genetics: A Quick Course

"We wish to suggest a structure for the salt of deoxyribose nucleic acid (D.N.A.). This structure has novel features which are of considerable biological interest."

—James D. Watson and Francis H. Crick
—Nature, April 25, 1953

With that masterly stroke of understatement, Watson and Crick, two gawky young scientists racing their colleagues in a Cambridge laboratory, ushered in the era of molecular biology. In 1968, when he published *The Double Helix*, Watson pondered how they unraveled the twisted strand of life, the winding DNA molecule. During those feverish years in the early 50s, wrote Watson, DNA was a "mystery up for grabs."

The solution to that mystery has led, in rapid order, all the way to gene therapy. Scientists can now reach down into the smallest unit of life-giving instructions, and rewrite the code. It won't be long before they perfect this technique and apply the fix to all manner of diseases. At least that's the hope.

For now, let's go back to basics. This chapter will reacquaint you with genetics, and suggest ways you can explain it to patients, if asked, using understandable language and common analogies.

The Book of Life

For some, it may rob life of its romance to know we boil down to a handful of chemicals that direct everything we are. But those few chemicals—often called "letters" in the Book of Life—have a great deal to say when combined and strung together just so. Adenine, thymine, cytosine and guanine (A, T, C, G) make up our alphabet, building blocks of the original "body language." These bases form in pairs: A and T together

TABLE I

The Genetic Code

This is how the four chemical bases in mRNA combine into codons to produce the 20 amino acids. A = adenine, C = cytosine, U = uracil, G = guanine

UUU UUC **Translate into** **phenylalanine**	CAU CAC **Translate** **into histidine**	AAA AAG **Translate** **into lysine**
UCU UCC UCA UCG AGU AGC **Translate into serine**	CAA CAG **Translate** **into glycine**	GUU GUC GUA GUG **Translate** **into valine**
UAU UAC **Translate** **into tyrosine**	CGU CGC CGA CGG AGA AGG **Translate** **into arginine**	GCU GCC GCA GCG **Translate** **into alanine**
UGU UGC **Translate** **into cysteine**	AUU AUC AUA **Translate** **into isoleucine**	GAU GAC **Translate into** **aspartic acid**
UGG **Translates** **into tryptophan**	AUG **Translates** **into methionine**	GAA GAG **Translate into** **glutamine**
UUA UUG CUU CUC CUA CUG **Translate** **into leucine**	ACU ACC ACA ACG **Translate** **into threonine**	GGU GGC GGA GGG **Translate into** **glutamic acid**
CCU CCC CCA CCG **Translate** **into proline**	AAU AAC **Translate into** **asparagine**	**STOP** **CODONS** **UAA** **UGA** **UAG**

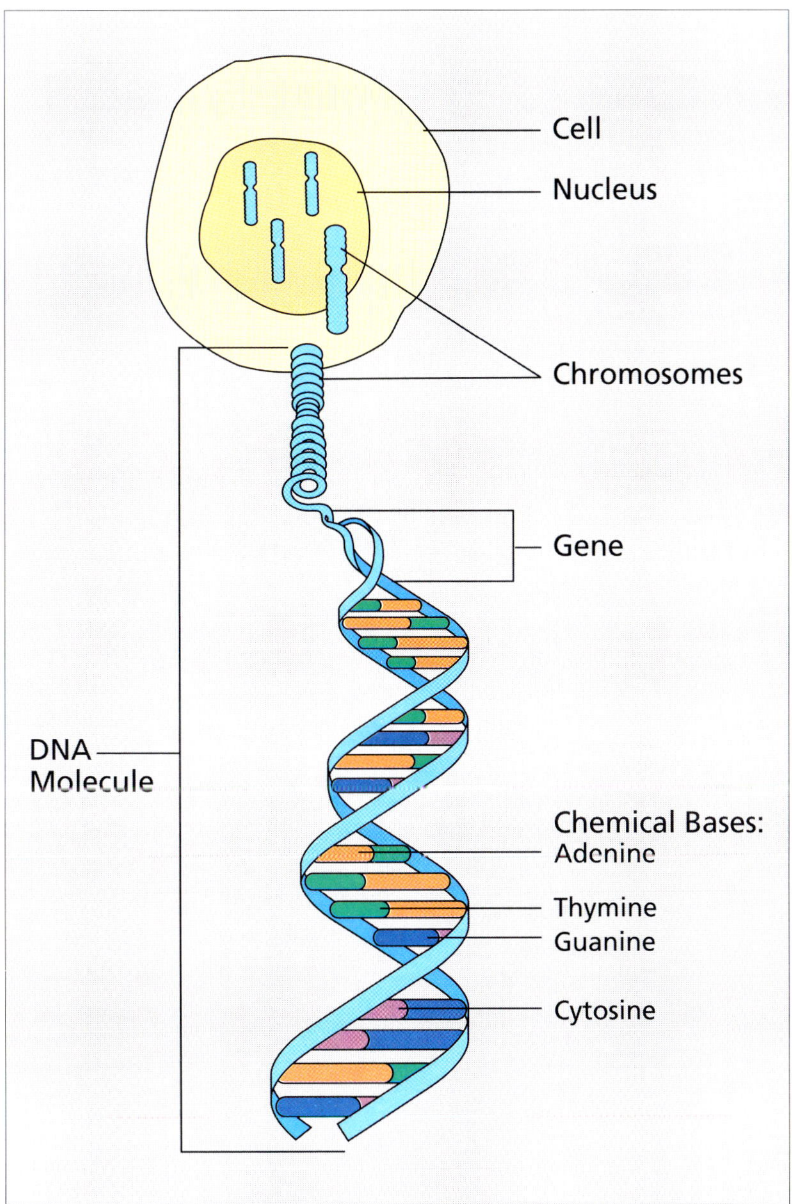

Figure 1: Double Helix—DNA, which carries the instructions that allow cells to make proteins, is made up of four chemical bases. Tightly coiled strands of DNA are packaged in our chromosomes, housed in the cell's nucleus. Genes are the working subunits of DNA.

forever, C and G, likewise. They are the most important part of DNA.

It took an astronomer, George Gamow, to suggest that these four chemical bases could combine in groups of three to cook up amino acids. The three-letter groups, or codons, serve as the "words" in the Book of Life. In the 1960s the Indian biochemist Har Gobind Khorana figured out the 64 possible codons and the 20 amino acids they specify. For instance, ACG creates threonine; GAG codes for glutamine. When strung together the amino acids produce the blueprint for proteins built by the body's cells. Hormones, enzymes, and antibodies—these are all examples of proteins vital to the structure, function, and regulation of the body.

Codons make up our 100,000 genes—"sentences" in the DNA Book of Life. To the untrained eye, the string of codons looks like a long line of babble. Where do the sentences start and end? It turns out that three "stop codons" signal the end of each gene, UAA, UGA, and UAG (See Table 1).

As in any book, the sentences fit into chapters—in this case, our 46 chromosomes, dwelling in the nucleus of every somatic cell in the body—altogether 22 pairs of autosomes and 2 sex chromosomes (XX in women; XY in men). Sex cells—sperm and egg—contain 23 chromosomes; when the two halves combine during mating, the full complement of chromosomes come together. The word chromosome comes from the Greek words *chroma*, meaning "color," and "*soma*," meaning body. In the 19th century, scientists knew that if they dyed dividing cells, they could stain the chromosomes' threadlike protein structures within.

When stained and viewed under a powerful light microscope today, chromosomes reveal a pattern of light and dark bands. These bands indicate variations in the amounts of nucleotides—that is, the four bases plus their attached sugars and phosphates (see Figure 1). (Thymine substitutes for uracil in DNA). The differences allow researchers to distinguish the chromosomes from one another in an analysis called a karyotype (see Figure 2). It's important to categorize the chromosomes in this way when searching for the exact location of specific genes, or for mutations—missing, broken or extra

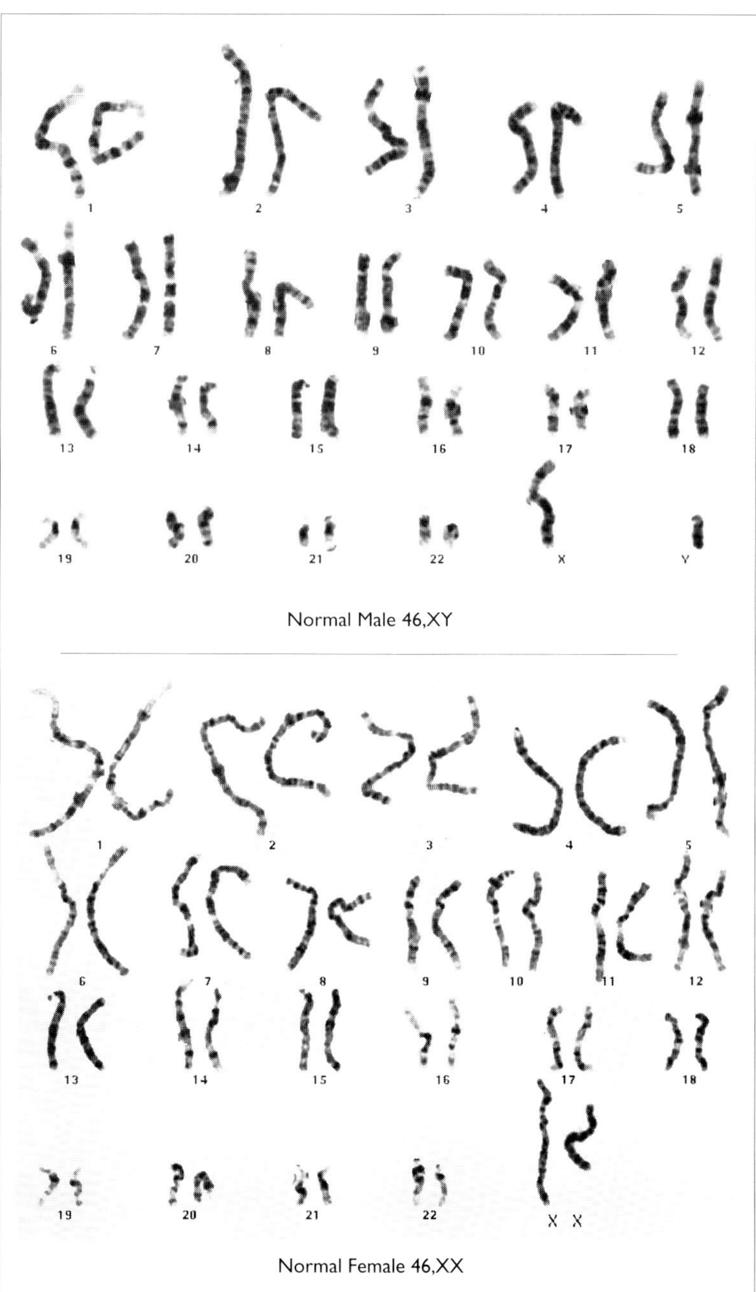

Figure 2: Each person's 23 pairs of human chromosomes can be distinguished by size and by unique banding patterns.

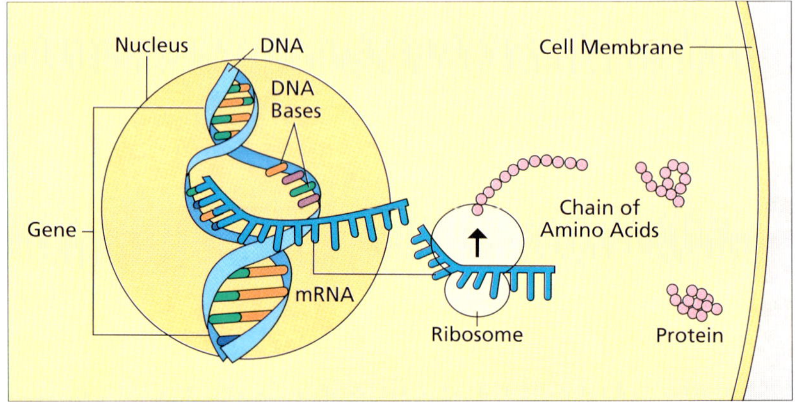

Figure 3: For a cell to make a protein, the information from a gene is copied, base by base, from DNA into new strands of messenger RNA (mRNA). Then mRNA travels out of the nucleus into the cysoplasm, to cell organeles called ribosomes. There mRNA directs the assembly of amino acids that fold into a completed protein molecule.

copies of a chromosome. People with Down's syndrome, for instance, have a third copy of chromosome 21.

The Double Helix

When Watson and Crick offered up their twisting ladder of life, they dryly observed, "It has not escaped our notice that the specific pairing we have postulated immediately suggests a possible copying mechanism for the genetic material." In fact,

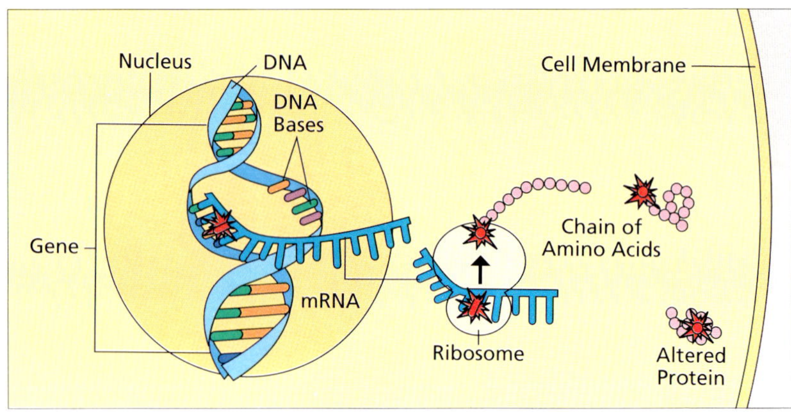

Figure 4: When a gene contains a mutation, the protein encoded by that gene will be abnormal. Some protein changes are insignificant, others are disabling.

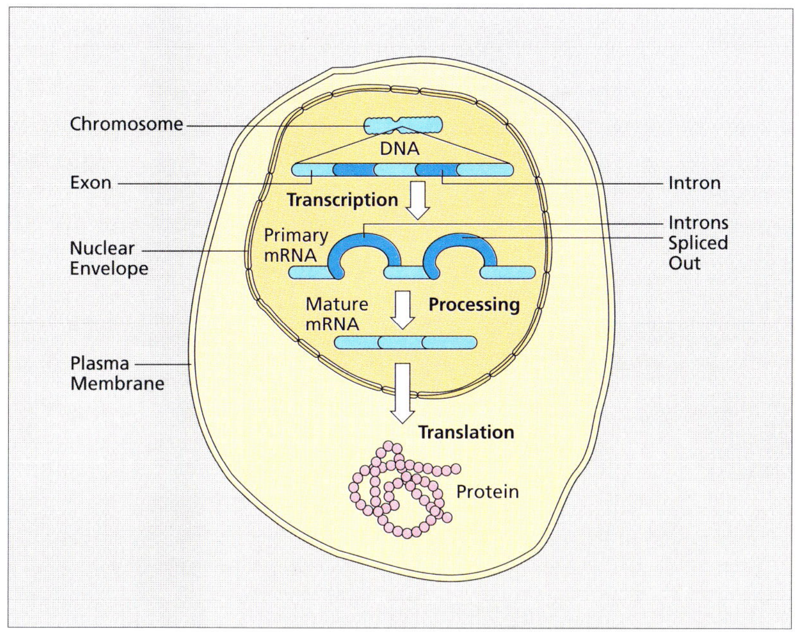

Figure 5: A summary of the steps leading from DNA to proteins. Replication and transcription occur in the cell nucleus, after which then mRNA is transported to the cytoplasm, where translation of the mRNA into amino acid sequences composing a protein occurs.

you can't help but feel awed by the elegance of this information-storing, self-replicating molecule tightly coiled in our cells. It means that like can beget like; the world can keep turning.

How does it happen? Let's look first at the makeup of DNA. We've already talked about the four most important components: the bases adenine and thymine, cytosine and guanine. They comprise the rungs of the ladder, paired and held together by weak hydrogen bonds. Sugar (deoxyribose) and phosphate serve as the ladder's uprights. When a gene puts in an order for a protein, the two uprights tear away, "unzipping" the molecule (Figure 3), leaving each base unpaired. Watson and Crick's postulated "specific pairing" dictates that the partner-less bases will always attract their complementary opposite. That means that at the end of DNA's day, a new double-stranded molecule, identical to the original, will have formed.

Enzymes help move this process along. One enzyme unravels the double helix, another holds the strands apart, and another—DNA polymerase—plays a key role in replication. Like a good referee, polymerase makes sure everyone plays by the rules, seeing that adenine, for instance, doesn't wander into guanine's berth or cytosine hasn't encroached on thymine's turf. Polymerase corrects such mistakes, shooing off the interlopers and waving in the proper base. If polymerase fails to blow the whistle, mutations occur (Figure 4), and that could lead to genetic diseases.

Once new DNA has formed in the nucleus, the cell's head office, protein synthesis can take place. But someone has to go out into the cytoplasm, the cell's workfloor, and inform the machine shop workers, the ribosomes, that it's time to assemble the amino acids and proteins. That "someone" is RNA: ribonucleic acid, a single-strand molecule chemically similar to DNA, except for its ribose sugar and its uracil base (U), which can stand in for thymine. As the executive assistant, RNA must perform two duties: transcribe and translate DNA's instructions.

To transcribe (Figure 5), RNA calls into action its own polymerase enzyme which hitches on to a DNA site at the beginning of a gene. The RNA polymerase then pulls a section of the DNA strand apart to expose unattached DNA bases. One of these loose DNA strands acts as a template for the messenger or "mRNA." Before the nucleus deems this transcripted message mature enough for release, the head office gives mRNA a once-over. Nuclear enzymes snip out noncoding sections called introns (the enigmatic "junk DNA") and splice together other sections called exons, the working sequences that code for proteins. (There's room for error here: if the gene splicing goes awry, mutations can appear.) Now ready to convey, or translate DNA's instructions, the mRNA bustles out of the nucleus into the cytoplasm.

Inherit the Blend

Genes come in pairs, one from each parent. Gregor Mendel, the 19th century Austrian monk so fascinated by peas, came up with the notion of paired factors or "elements" as he called

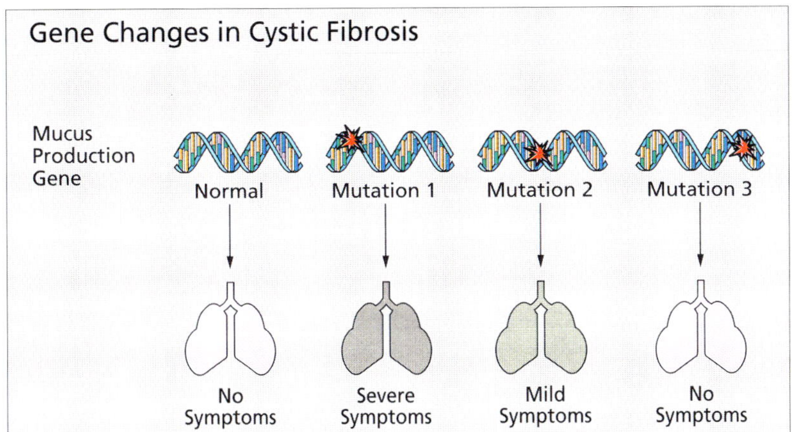

Figure 6: Different mutations in the same gene can produce a wide range of effects. In cystic fibrosis, for instance, the gene that controls mucus production can have more than 300 different mutations; some cause severe symptoms; some, mild symptoms; and some, no symptoms at all.

them. Today we call these elements alleles, one of two or more forms of the same gene. Of each pair, one is often dominant, meaning that it masks the other. Mendel found this out by observing what happened when he crossed tall pea plants with short plants, and plants with different colored flowers. The masked, or recessive allele doesn't disappear, he discovered; it can show up in a later generation.

In the case of human eye color, one allele produces brown eyes, another makes blue eyes. Your gene pair for eye color may be:
• Blue/Blue, making you homozygous with respect to that gene, and blue-eyed;
• Brown/Brown making you homozygous and brown-eyed; or
• Brown/Blue which means you are heterozygous but still brown-eyed, because the brown allele is dominant.

This explains why two parents with brown eyes, if they are both heterozygous, can produce blue-eyed children. (Note that modifier genes can alter these two colors to produce hazel, green, gray or even—improbably—violet eyes.)

While the system of inheritance works well to pass along such traits, it also can perpetuate mutations that lead to trouble. Considering that 3 billion DNA base pairs replicate in

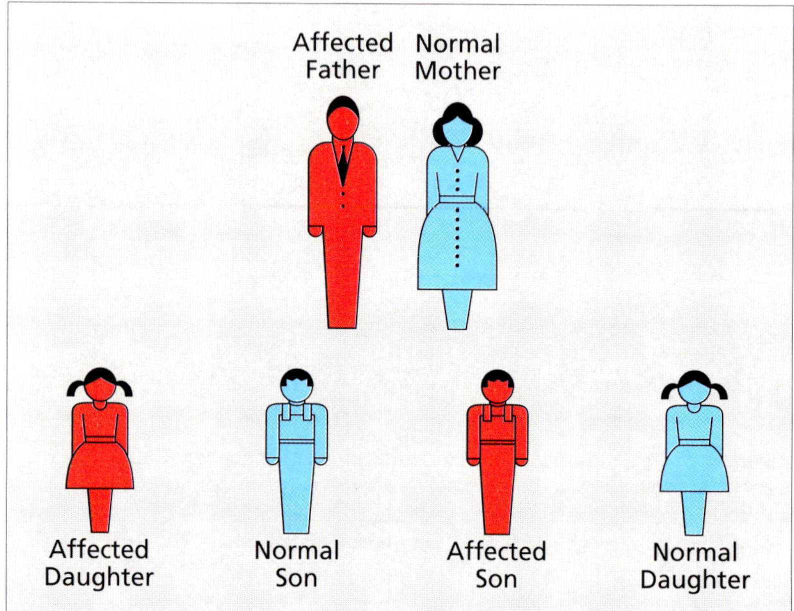

Figure 7: In dominant genetic disorders, if one affected parent has a disease-causing allele that dominates its normal counterpart, each child in the family has a 50% chance of inheriting the disease allele and the disorder.

each cell division, the process is amazingly accurate. Scientists estimate that the proofreading and repair team—several dozen enzymes—mop up 99.9% of errors. Yet misspellings do slip through. And the simplest misprint can have the most drastic consequences. For example, our oxygen-toting protein, hemoglobin, consists of a string of 146 amino acids. If even one amino acid in that chain—valine—seizes the rightful spot of another—glutamic acid—the entire protein malfunctions. It's just a small typo: GAA changed to GUA, a point mutation. But it's enough to cause sickle cell anemia. Other types of mutation: deletions or insertions. They can produce extra or missing amino acids in a protein and hence defective genes. Many cases of cystic fibrosis, for instance, result from a three-base pair deletion (see Figure 6).

Inherited genetic diseases result from DNA flawed in the

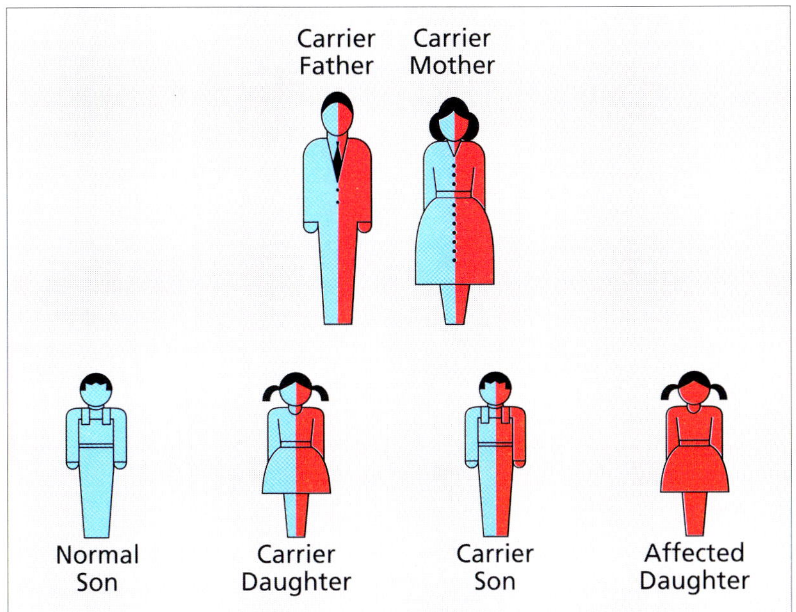

Figure 8: In diseases associated with altered recessive genes, both parents—though disease-free themselves—carry one normal allele and one altered allele. Each child has one chance in four of inheriting two normal alleles; and two chances in four of inheriting one normal and one altered allele, and being a carrier like both parents. Examples of recessive disorders, albeit rare, which predispose to breast cancer are ataxia telangiectasia and Bloom's Syndrome.

sex, or germline, cells. These blunders can pass from one generation to the next in three ways:

• *Autosomal dominant*, in which the defective gene need be present in only one (dominant) allele in order for the disease to show outwardly (see Figure 7).

• *Autosomal recessive*, in which the defective (recessive) gene must be inherited in a double dose to cause abnormality. Parents can carry masked copies of the recessive gene without having the disease themselves. But when two such parents mate and pass along two copies of the masked gene, the disease reveals itself in their child (see Figure 8).

• *X-linked recessive*, in which a disease that is caused by a defect in the X chromosome usually leads to illness in males in whom the defect cannot be masked by a second, normal X chromosome.

Nature Plus Nurture

While errors in somatic cells may cause disease, including some cancers, they don't carry forward to the next generation. That makes these diseases genetic but not inherited events. In fact, most cancers arise in this way. Tripped perhaps by too much sun exposure, a close encounter with toxic chemicals, or faulty DNA repair, sometimes genes stumble, forcing somatic mutations.

Over time genetic mistakes accumulate in the body's tissues and random or "sporadic" cancers can take root with cells proliferating unchecked. Oncologists tag this "deregulation." In revolt, the cells have chucked out the rule book on when to stop growing and when to start differentiating into specialized units. Essentially, there are two types of genes that jump-start this revolt:

Tumor-suppressor genes. Under normal conditions these genes act as brakes on cell growth. When missing or inactivated, the brakes fail and a malignant bloom can veer out of control. Among the most notorious of the tumor-suppressor genes is p53, involved in transcription and cell cycle regulation. When p53 turns bad, it turns very bad, responsible for breast and colon cancers, leukemia, and soft tissue sarcomas, among others. Mutant versions of p53 have been found in DNA samples from more than half of human tumors, making it the most common gene linked with cancer. Other examples of tumor suppressors: APC which causes colon, pancreatic and stomach cancers; RB which causes retinoblastoma, osteosarcoma, breast, lung, prostate and bladder cancers; and WT1 which causes nephroblastoma (Wilms' tumor).

Oncogenes. Normally these genes accelerate cell growth (in a controlled way). When mutated or "over"-activated, the oncogene accelerator gets stuck to the floor, flooding cells with signals that shout: "Keep on dividing!" The end result: a high-speed, wild cellular ride—essentially the same outcome as if the tumor-suppressor brakes had failed. Some examples of oncogenes: RAF, which leads to stomach cancer; MYC, which leads to lymphomas; and TRK which leads to thyroid tumors. In a number of colon cancers, pathologists have found activated RAS oncogenes living side-by-side with inactivated tumor-

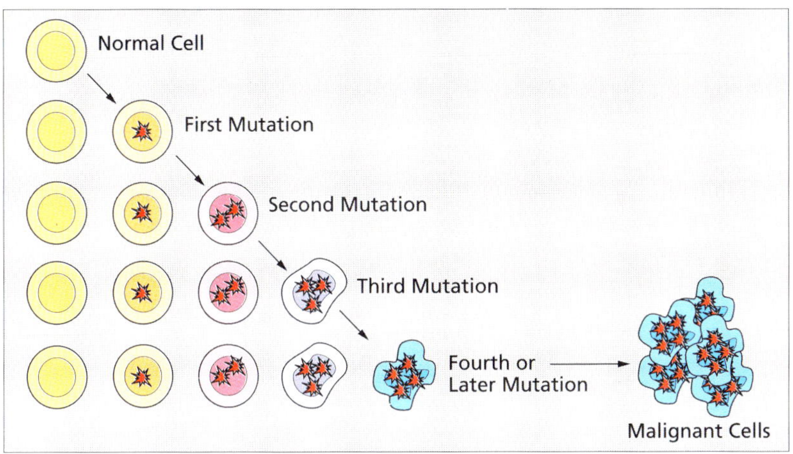

Figure 9: Cancer usually arises in a single cell. The cell's progress from normal to malignant to metastatic appears to follow a series of distinct steps, each controlled by a different gene or set of genes. Persons with hereditary cancer already have the first mutation.

suppressor genes such as p53. This suggests that creating cancer may require *both* types of genetic changes.

So far, we've been referring to these mutations in somatic cells. But they can take place in germline cells as well, which means that cancer-causing genes can pass to offspring, producing families with a large number of breast, ovarian, or colon cancers, for example. Such "cancer families" are rare, but that's cold comfort to those who inherit the mutant allele that leads to a tumor. However, we don't inherit cancer so much as a *predisposition* to cancer. It takes a confluence of events from within the body and without (Figure 9) to produce pathology. Nature (genes) and nurture (diet, mutagenic environmental exposure) each play a role. This means that even though genes may dictate what we are, by changing a harmful lifestyle we can better control what we become.

An oft-cited example: In Japan, the lifetime risk of colon cancer was ten times lower than in the United States: 0.5% versus 5%. Epidemiologists who studied Japanese immigrants to the US found that among the first-generation Japanese living in Hawaii, the frequency of colon cancer rose several fold: not as high as on the US mainland, but higher than in Japan. By the time second-generation Japanese had lived on the mainland, their colon cancer rates equaled that of other Americans. All this implicated diet and lifestyle as important factors in the development of disease.

But that doesn't mean genetic factors play no role. Some North Americans still contract colon cancers while others do not. How does research account for that? Differences within the environment such as varied diet, and differences in genetic predisposition. (For instance, when a first degree relative has colon cancer, an individual's risk rises several fold.) And how did scientists account for the difference in colon cancer frequency between Japanese living in their native country and immigrants to the US? One theory: something in the Asian environment rendered the predisposing genes less penetrant— that is, less likely to result in disease.

Gene Hunters

In both real estate and genetics, it seems, location is everything. Knowing where on the chromosomes human genes reside will forever change medical practice and biomedical research. With the genetic blueprint in hand, we can better understand how humans develop from a single cell, how genes govern the functions of tissues and organs, how the disease process devolves. And that will lead to better diagnosis, treatment, and even prevention of disease.

Toward these ends, the federal government established the National Center for Human Genome Research (NCHGR) in 1989. This center directs the United States' role in the Human Genome Project, a gargantuan effort to decipher our DNA— the Book of Life, the genome. On 25 October 1996, the journal *Science* published a partially complete gene map compiled by an international team of 100 scientists. The map, which you can explore at the interactive Internet site www.ncbi.nlm.nih.gov/SCIENCE96/, nails down the location of one-fifth of our genes.

Francis S. Collins, MD, PhD, who heads the NCHGR, pioneered a powerful gene-finding method known as "positional cloning" that has given an enormous boost to genome mapping. The technique has isolated dozens of disease genes including those for retinoblastoma, Wilms' tumor, Von Hippel-

Lindau disease, breast and ovarian cancers. To isolate and clone such target genes, the Collins technique relies on other potent tools that sift through the genome haystack of 3 billion base pairs. As scientists hone these tools and tie them together, they drive the gene hunt forward faster and cheaper. At the beginning of the gene pursuit it took months—sometimes years—and $5 to find each base pair; now it costs only weeks of time and as little as 50¢ per nucleotide by using improved methods of:

Genetic (or Linkage) Mapping. This is the first step in isolating a gene, and offers firm evidence that a disease or trait is linked to a culprit gene (or genes) passed from parent to child. Genetic mapping also provides clues about which chromosome contains the gene and where on that chromosome the gene lies. Using blood or tissue samples from members of a family in which a disease occurs, scientists first isolate DNA from the samples. They then look for markers—characteristic

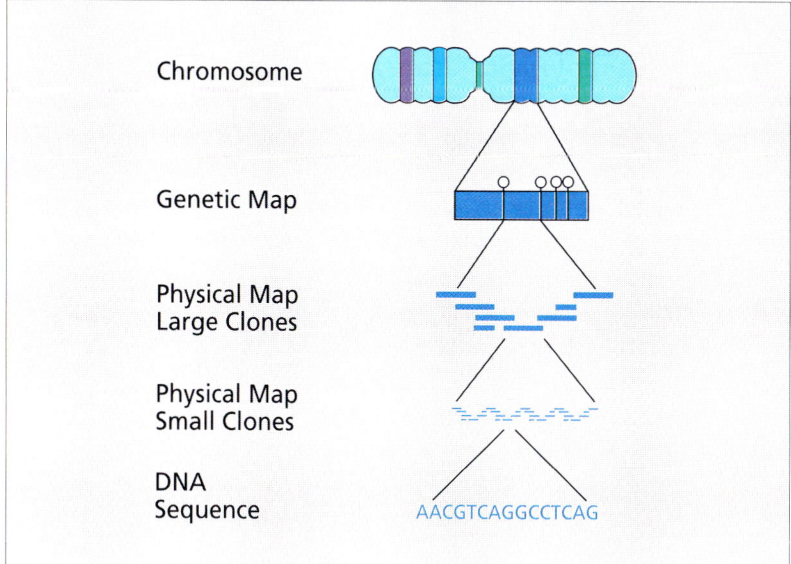

Figure 10: Maps of DNA can have several levels of detail: from the banding patterns of the chromosomes, to clones of overlapping segments of DNA, and ultimately to the base-by-base sequence of DNA.

molecular patterns inherited along with the disease, piggy-back fashion. The more markers on the map, the more likely one of them will relate to a disease gene, making it much easier for researchers to zero in on the gene.

Markers consist of slight spelling differences in the genetic alphabet A, T, C, and G. Called "polymorphisms," these differences usually occur in the so-called junk DNA and normally do not affect a person's health. But they can tell a researcher from whom the DNA came, making them useful in tracking inheritance through generations. Police departments and coroners also use such DNA "fingerprints" to identify victims and perpetrators.

In 1994 an international group of investigators published a genetic map with nearly 6,000 markers spaced, on average, less than a million bases apart. Leaders of the Human Genome Project announced that the map contains more details than originally hoped for, and was completed a full year ahead of schedule. Since then, scientists have continued to fine-tune this map.

Physical Mapping. Once scientists use genetic mapping to assign a gene to a small area on a chromosome, they must then examine that region more closely to find the gene's exact location for a physical map. To construct such a map, gene hunters use restriction enzymes—nature's scissors—to slice apart a chromosome into smaller, workable pieces. They then copy, or clone, the pieces, matching them up in their starting order so they can trace the origin and genetic content of each one. The data go into a computer, and the DNA snippets into a freezer. When a genetic linkage map shows that a gene lies in a certain region, it narrows the search for the gene in question. Next step: defrost and examine the appropriate copied pieces. They should lead to another gene and a new entry on the physical map.

Because it's essential to keep track of the chromosome pieces in their proper order, scientists had to develop a system of markers much like the mile posts on a highway. In this case the markers connect one section of chromosome "road" with the next. Cloned pieces of DNA road overlap in places that share the same marker (called "sequenced-tagged site"). These mile post markers let researchers know how far they have driven along the chromosome to their destination—the disease gene they seek. With few markers to guide them in the past, scientists used to spend as many as 10 years traveling lonely stretches of chromosome highway searching in vain for a gene.

The original goal for sets of overlapping DNA pieces, or "contigs," was that they measure 2 million bases in length by 1995. By 1996 the contigs ranged from 20 million to 50 million bases. Already, researchers have pieced together enough sets to complete chromosomes 21, 22, and Y, and nearly all of chromosomes 3, 4, 7, 11, 12, 16, 19, and X. The ultimate goal: every chromosome in the human genome.

DNA Sequencing. Physical maps provide the raw material for understanding the sequence of bases—the four essential letters—A, T, C and G—in the Book of Life. By knowing the correct sequence of these letters and the genes that they compose, scientists can spot the specific aberrations that may cause disease.

To construct the human genome, scientists find it useful to sequence other organisms used in research as models for human disease: *E. coli*, the gut bacterium; *C. elegans*, a microscopic see-through roundworm; drosophila (fruit flies); and mice. In the spring of 1996 researchers completed the sequence for baker's yeast, significant because yeast resembles human cells more closely than do bacteria. Because of their relative simplicity, these organisms make an ideal testing ground for new sequencing technology.

For example, labs working on the roundworm *C. elegans* have increased their annual production rate to 15 million base pairs. (With 100 million base pairs to sequence in the worm, researchers expect to finish by 1998.) During the 1970s, labs could barely churn out a few base pairs per year, hardly up to the task of tackling 3 billion. When the Human Genome Project got underway in 1990, few labs had sequenced even 100,000 bases. Since then, improved technology and automation have increased speed and lowered cost considerably. Genome project officials feel quite certain that they can reach the goal of sequencing the entire human genome by the year 2003.

Delivering the Promise

In 2003, when the Human Genome Project crosses the finish line after 15 years and billions of dollars, this Big Science effort will signal more of a beginning than an end. The genome "provides grist for the next generations of effort to figure out how the genes work," says Dr. Collins. But patients want more than just the promise of the human genome—they want their disease treated, cured. And eventually that will come.

For now, says Dr. Collins, gene testing affords doctors the chance to practice "individualized preventive medicine in which they focus medical surveillance and lifestyle management on the people who need it most." It's unrealistic to think that gene therapies will be on the market in the next few years, he points out. But finding disease genes puts us that much closer.

In Chapters 3, 4, and 5 we will address some of the most-asked questions about cancers for which researchers have pinned down some of the culprit genes: breast, ovarian, colon, Von Hippel-Lindau, retinoblastoma, Wilms', and thyroid. (Bear in mind, however, that most patients *do not* inherit these cancers; they occur at random.) We also provide a list of resources.

CHAPTER 3

The Genetics of Breast and Ovarian Cancer

"It's always something."

—*Gilda Radner, Comedian*
Felled by hereditary ovarian cancer

W**hat are the genes associated with hereditary breast and ovarian cancers?**
Mutations in at least five genes predispose women to breast cancer: mutations on BRCA1, BRCA2, p53 (associated with Li-Fraumeni Syndrome), CD1 (associated with Cowden Syndrome), and possibly ATM (ataxia telangiectasia mutated). Research will probably uncover other genes as well. We all carry every one of these genes, mostly in their normal form. They can mutate in hundreds or even thousands of ways, some alterations are unique to a given family. Mutations often crop up at "hot spots"—areas of the gene where scientists have found more than one genetic flaw.

Women who inherit a mutated form of the genes BRCA1 or BRCA2 have as much as a 90% lifetime chance of developing breast cancer, and as much as a 60% chance of developing ovarian cancer during their lifetime. Researchers reckon that these genes account for 5% to 10% of all such cancers, as well as an excess number of colon and prostate cancers—about three times as many as occur in the general population. When linked to BRCA1 and BRCA2, breast and ovarian cancers strike early—in a woman's 40s on average as opposed to her 60s as you might expect with sporadic forms of these diseases. Mutations in BRCA2 also are associated with rare male breast cancer.

In October 1996, investigators at Memorial Sloan-Kettering Cancer Center reported that a specific alteration in the BRCA2 gene is just as common as a BRCA1 mutation among Jewish

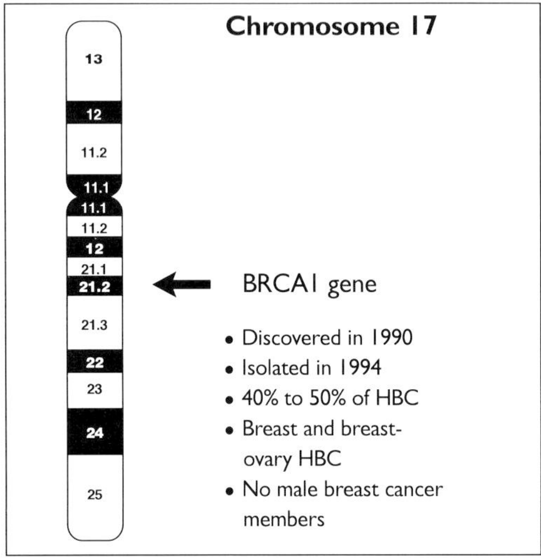

Figure 1: Location of the BRCA1 gene on chromosome 17. HBC=hereditary breast cancer

women of Eastern European descent, a group that includes more than 90% of the 6 million Jews living in the United States. However, the risk of breast cancer in this ethnic group is more than three times higher in women who inherit the BRCA1 mutation compared to those who inherit the BRCA2 mutation.

The study's lead author, Kenneth Offit, MD, expressed surprise, saying he expected the cancer risk of the two faulty genes to be about the same. According to Dr. Offit, about one in every 50 Ashkenazi Jews carries one of the two altered genes, "a frequency that is quite high," he says. The new estimates predict that, compared with the general population, the risk of early-onset breast cancer (before age 42) is 31 times greater in Ashkenazi women with the BRCA1 error, and 9 times greater than in those with the BRCA2 error.

In their normal guise, BRCA1 (found on chromosome 17) and BRCA2 (found on chromosome 13) appear to act as tu-

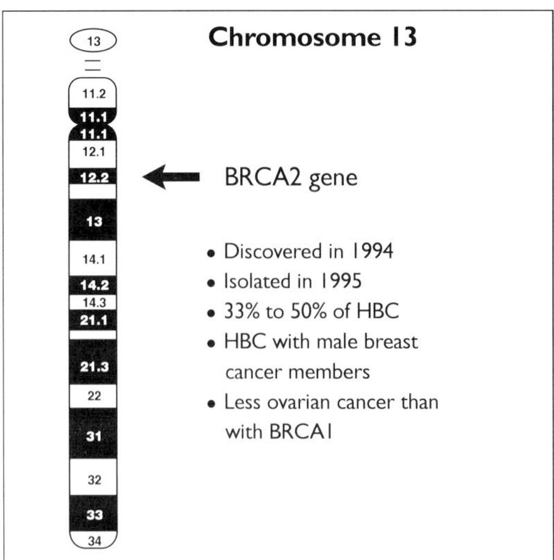

Figure 2: Location of the BRCA2 gene on chromosome 13. HBC=hereditary breast cancer

mor suppressor genes. So far, investigators have found more than 100 different mutations in BRCA1. One common gene flaw, especially among Ashkenazi Jews: what researchers call the "185delAG" gene. Translation: At codon number 185, the chemical bases adenine and guanine have been deleted. This DNA error cripples the gene's ability to code for a protein that places a brake on unchecked cell growth. In similar fashion BRCA2 can mutate in many ways; one variety is the "6174delT" mutation in which thymine has quit the scene at codon number 6174. Beyond that, researchers know few details.

Ironically, and oddly, a small study at the University of Pennsylvania recently showed that ovarian cancer patients with mutated BRCA1 genes lived longer than other such patients without the altered gene. And in Scandinavia, women with altered BRCA1 genes exhibited somewhat less deadly forms of breast cancer.

During the late 1960s and early 1970s, Henry Lynch, MD, and his colleagues at Creighton University and the National Cancer Institute, first described a hereditary breast-ovarian cancer syndrome. By studying the Hall family (see Chapter 7), and many others, Dr. Lynch was able to verify how both breast and ovarian cancer fit into an autosomal dominant inheritance pattern. In certain members of the Hall family, patients were diagnosed with both types of cancer; in other cases a mother with ovarian cancer produced daughters who developed breast or ovarian cancer or both. Likewise, some mothers with breast cancer gave rise to daughters with breast or ovarian cancer or both.

What other risk factors predispose patients to breast and ovarian cancers?

Certainly, the more first-degree relatives struck by cancer, the higher one's chances of contracting the disease. But often it takes more than wayward genes alone to create tumors.

Risk factors for breast cancer include:
- Early menstruation (before age 12) or late menopause (after age 55)
- First pregnancy after age 30 or nulliparity
- Tallness (linked to a slightly higher risk for premenopausal

breast cancer) and obesity (linked to a higher risk for breast cancer after age 50)

- Alcohol consumption
- Use of estrogen (still controversial)

Also under study: the connection between breast cancer and high-fat diet; smoking; lack of exercise; exposure to pesticides, engine exhausts, contaminants in food and water; abortion; miscarriage; choosing not to breast-feed.

Risk factors under investigation for ovarian cancer include:

- High-fat diet
- Use of talc (an asbestos-related product that can reach the ovaries through the cervix) in the genital area
- No pregnancies or infertility
- Use of fertility-stimulating drugs that induce ovulation and create more disruption to ovarian tissue

Can prophylactic surgeries prevent hereditary breast and ovarian cancers?

Even though some women have taken this step, we need more research to answer that question definitively. It seems logical: remove the ovaries, for instance, and you cut out the cancer risk. The problem: ovarian tissue derives from the same embryonic cells as the peritoneum. Among women who opt for oophorectomy, 3% to 5% contract an ovarian cancer-like pathology in the peritoneal tissue. But that risk must be viewed in perspective and compared with the 40% to 66% lifetime ovarian cancer risk for a BRCA1 mutation carrier.

Removing the ovaries before natural menopause creates an abrupt loss of estrogen production. That can lead to such side effects as dry vagina as well as an increased lifetime risk for osteoporosis and heart disease. Hormone replacement therapy (both estrogen and progestin) could ease these side effects. But controversy remains on whether estrogen increases the risk for breast cancer.

Unfortunately, early detection of ovarian cancers has proved exceedingly difficult, even with high-tech transvaginal ovarian ultrasound and the CA-125 blood test. In most cases, by the time doctors detect the disease it has progressed to an inoperable, incurable stage. Once women understand the limitations of available screening techniques, some may view prophylactic oophorectomy as a more acceptable choice.

According to studies conducted at M.D. Anderson Cancer Center, prophylactic mastectomies appear to offer greater protection against cancer than oophorectomies. Among 3,000 patients with a family history of breast cancer who had had preventive mastectomies, only 1% of the 800 highest risk patients developed the disease after surgery. While surgeons cannot remove *all* the breast tissue, it appears that with less tissue left behind, less chance remains for disease to evolve.

Of course, physicians have found more success in screening for breast cancer than ovarian cancer. Mammography tends to work better among women over 50 whose fattier breasts yield their inner landscape more readily. But the x-rays cannot always detect cancers early enough in younger women whose denser breast tissue can cloak tiny tumors. Despite that, Dr. Lynch recommends that women at inordinately high risk for hereditary breast cancer begin screening at age 25, repeating the procedure every other year through age 35, and then annually thereafter. Such caution is warranted, he says, because so many of these women will contract breast cancer in their mid-40s. And for those facing heritable disease, prophylactic surgery starts to look like an option, if an uncertain one.

Where can patients and doctors turn for more help?
For sources of further information and counseling/testing for your patients, see Appendix 1 and Appendix 2.

CHAPTER 4

The Genetics of Colon Cancer

*"Genetic research like this would have been
science fiction 10 years ago."*

*—Bert Vogelstein, MD
Howard Hughes Medical Institute
Johns Hopkins Oncology Center*

What are the genes associated with hereditary
colon cancer?
Researchers have identified two main forms of hereditary colon cancer: familial adenomatous polyposis (many
colonic polyps), or FAP; and hereditary nonpolyposis colorectal
cancer, or HNPCC (few if any polyps). FAP represents less
than 1% of all colorectal cancer cases doctors diagnose each
year; HNPCC perhaps 5% to 10%. Most colon cancers occur
sporadically, or cluster in susceptible families (see Figure 1).

FAP arises from mutations in the APC (adenomatous
polyposis coli) gene on chromosome 5, a gene normally meant
to inhibit cell growth. With the brakes off, hundreds or even
thousands of adenomatous polyps can form in the colon by the
time an affected child reaches 16. Some patients develop these
polyps by the time they turn 10; nearly all do by age 35. Most
of the polyps measure less than 5 mm in diameter, growing so
thickly they carpet the entire colon surface. Unless surgeons
remove the colon, cancer inevitably strikes. By the time FAP
patients see their doctors (usually complaining of diarrhea,
abdominal pain, or rectal bleeding) two-thirds have already
developed cancer. Many FAP patients also develop a number
of gastric polyps that rarely cause colon cancer or other
problems. But other cancers can strike these patients, including periampullary carcinoma, gastric cancer, thyroid, and
brain tumors. In 5% of patients, the trauma of surgery can
lead to desmoid tumors.

HNPCC arises from mutations in any one of four genes

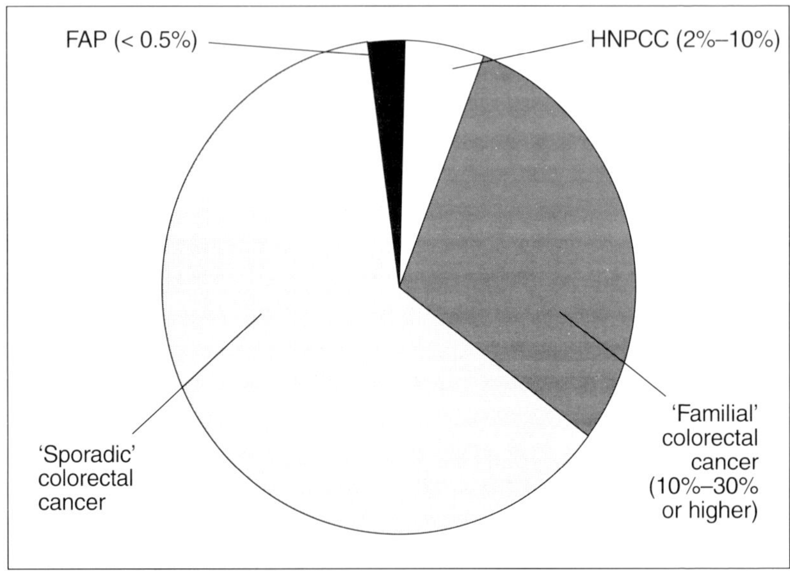

Figure 1: Causes of colorectal cancer

meant to repair "mismatches" between reconstituted base pairs. Two of these genes reside on chromosome 2, one on chromosome 3, and the fourth on chromosome 7. Different families carry different faulty genes.

The mismatch errors force mutations to accumulate in tumor suppressor genes and oncogenes, mistakes that eventually lead to cancer. Usually by the time an affected person reaches age 45, he or she will develop colorectal cancer with only one or a few adenomatous polyps present.

Most clinicians and cancer geneticists would agree that certain cardinal clinical features characterize HNPCC. These include the following: autosomal dominant inheritance pattern; gene penetrance of approximately 85% to 90%; early age of CRC onset ($\approx$ age 45); proximal colonic predilection to CRC ($\approx$ 70% proximal to the splenic flexure); and a significant excess of synchronous and metachronous CRC (46% metachronous CRC within 10 years following initial CRC when less than a subtotal colectomy has been performed). These features are consonant with the so-called Lynch syndrome I variant of HNPCC; in the case of Lynch syndrome II, all of these features are present but in addition patients have an inordinately increased susceptibility to certain extracolonic cancers, the most common of which is cancer of the endometrium, followed by carcinoma of the ovary, stomach, small bowel, pancreas, ureter, renal pelvis, and breast.

In the Lynch syndromes, some 70% of colon cancers appear in the right side of the colon. That means doctors must screen these patients with a full colonoscopy instead of flexible sigmoidosdcopy which only reaches the left side. These patients run an excess lifetime risk of colon cancer (85 to 90%). Since the entire colonic mucosa is susceptible to cancer it is especially important that the initial colon cancer surgery remove the entire colon. Leaving any segment behind puts the patient at a very high risk for recurrence.

What other risk factors predispose patients to colon cancer?

Research implicates a number of adverse lifestyle choices in sporadic cases of colon cancer: high fat, low fiber diet, little exercise, smoking, and alcohol overuse. How much these choices contribute to hereditary cancer remains unclear. Still, few would argue the overall health benefits of eating lots of fresh fruits and vegetables and grains, maintaining proper weight through regular exercise, reducing exposure to environmental toxins and tobacco.

What do experts recommend for surveillance and prevention?

FAP families

If an individual tests APC gene mutation positive:

• Starting around age 10 or 11, annual colon surveillance by flexible sigmoidoscopy.

• Prophylactic colectomy when numerous polyps appear. Preventive colectomy in the absence of polyps is *not* recommended.

• Surveillance for extracolonic neoplasms and periampullary carcinoma,especially upper GI tract adenomatous polyps.

If an individual tests APC gene mutation negative:

• At ages 18, 25, and 35 colon screening by flexible sigmoidoscopy.

• Because lifetime risk is the same as that of the general population, follow conventional screening guidelines.

HNPCC families
In at-risk family members:
• Colonoscopy every 2 years starting at age 20 to 25, and annually after age 35.
• Annual gynecologic exams in women with aspiration of endometrium for cytologic studies from age 30-35 onward.
• If doctors encounter other tumors in the family, screen for those tumors if a test is available, eg, upper endoscopy for small bowel tumors, urine cytology for urologic cancer.

In proven gene carriers:
• Same recommendations as for the at-risk family member, except colonoscopies are suggested every year starting at age 20-25, with the option of prophylactic colectomy.
In patients with colon cancer:
• Subtotal colectomy.
• Prophylactic hysterectomy and oophorectomy in women (after their family is completed) as an option, since screening for early onset ovarian cancer has serious limitations.
If doctors encounter other tumors in the family, screen for those tumors if a test is available.

Where can patients and doctors turn for more help?
Contact:
• Hereditary Cancer Institute, Creighton University School of Medicine, 2500 California Plaza, Omaha, NE 68178 (fax: 402-280-1734, phone: 402-280-2941)
• Hereditary Cancer Prevention Clinic, Attention Susan Tinley, RN, MS, 2500 California Plaza, Omaha, NE 68178 (fax: 402-280-1734; phone: 402-280-2942)
• Patrick M. Lynch, JD, MD; High Cancer Risk Clinic, M.D. Anderson Cancer Center, Division of GI Oncology, 1515 Holcombe Boulevard, Houston, TX 77030 (fax: 713-745-1163; phone: 713-792-2828)
• Johns Hopkins Oncology Center, 424 North Bond Street, Baltimore, MD 21231 (fax: 410-955-0548)

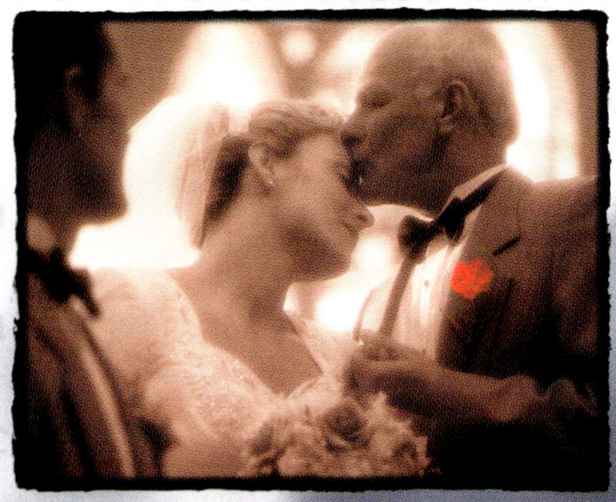

Give your patients a
survival advantage

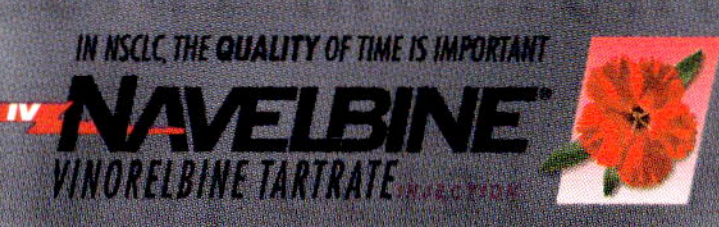

NAVELBINE plus cisplatin, in stages III and IV non-small cell lung cancer (NSCLC) as shown in large, randomized, well-controlled, multicenter studies...

- Unsurpassed one-year survival rates[1,2]
- Aggressive first-line therapy

Contraindicated in patients with pretreatment granulocyte counts <1,000 cells/mm.

Granulocytopenia is dose-limiting, but generally reversible and noncumulative over time.

References:
1. Le Chevalier T, Brisgand D, Douillard J-Y, et al. Randomized study of vinorelbine and cisplatin versus vindesine and cisplatin versus vinorelbine alone in advanced non-small cell lung cancer: results of a European multicenter trial including 612 patients. *J Clin Oncol.* 1994;12:360-367.
2. Data on file, Glaxo Wellcome Inc. [SWOG 9308 Phase III].

Please consult full Prescribing Information available at this exhibit.

GlaxoWellcome
Oncology/HIV
A division of Glaxo Wellcome Inc.
Research Triangle Park, NC 27709

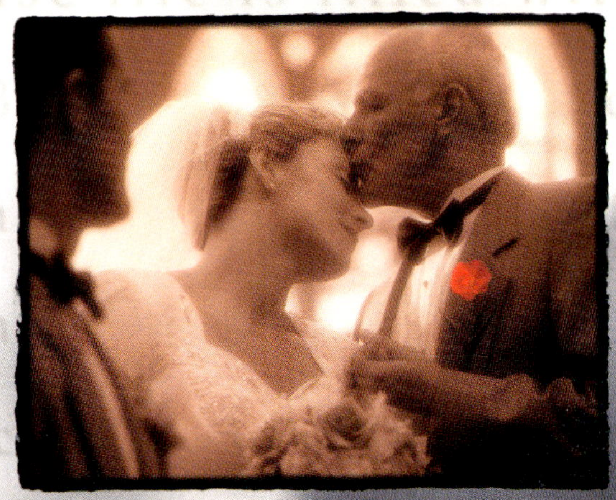

Give your patients a
survival advantage

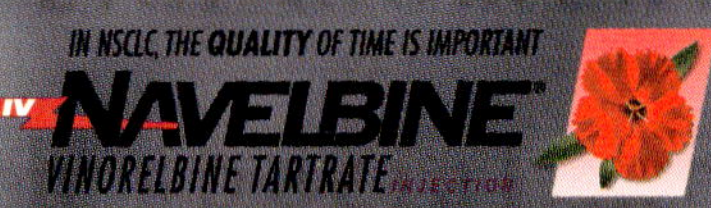

First-line—for performance and tolerability

NAVELBINE plus cisplatin, in stages III and IV non-small cell lung cancer (NSCLC) as shown in large, randomized, well-controlled, multicenter studies...

- Unsurpassed one-year survival rates[1,2]
- Aggressive first-line therapy

Contraindicated in patients with pretreatment granulocyte counts <1,000 cells/mm.

Granulocytopenia is dose-limiting, but generally reversible and noncumulative over time.

References:
1. Le Chevalier T, Brisgand D, Douillard J-Y, et al. Randomized study of vinorelbine and cisplatin versus vindesine and cisplatin versus vinorelbine alone in advanced non-small cell lung cancer: results of a European multicenter trial including 612 patients. *J Clin Oncol.* 1994;12:360-367.
2. Data on file, Glaxo Wellcome Inc. [SWOG 9308 Phase III].

Please consult full Prescribing Information available at this exhibit.

GlaxoWellcome
Oncology/HIV
A division of Glaxo Wellcome Inc.
Research Triangle Park, NC 27709

CHAPTER 5

The Rare Cancers

*"It's only rare when it happens
to someone else's family."*

—Parent of a child with retinoblastoma

W hile you may not encounter many cases of the more rare hereditary cancers, understanding retinoblastoma in particular sheds much light on how nature and nurture conspire to create cancer.

Retinoblastoma

Striking in roughly one out of every 20,000 births, these eye tumors begin during fetal development as retinal cells divide briskly. In nearly all cases, the disease manifests by age 5. Some 20% to 40% of retinoblastomas are hereditary; the rest occur sporadically. Scientists have traced the genetic abnormality to the RB gene on chromosome 13.

It was research on retinoblastoma that helped forge the link between inherited gene abnormalities and outside insults to somatic tissue—the landmark "two-hit" model of carcinogenesis offered by Alfred G. Knudson, MD, PhD, in 1971.* He reasoned that a second event could explain why, in a child who has inherited a mutant form of the RB gene, only a small fraction of the retinoblasts actually give rise to tumors. The first hit: a germline mutation. The second hit: probably the loss of marker DNA near the RB gene in the form of point mutations or deletions. The second hit removes the one good remaining allele of the gene. This implies that even when present in only a single copy, the RB gene can prevent tumor formation.

---

* In 1989 the American Cancer Society recognized Dr. Knudson's contribution with the
  Medal of Honor, its most prestigious award.

(Scientists originally coined the term "tumor suppressor" to describe this gene.)

For a sporadic case to occur, both mutations would have to take place independently in the same retinoblast—a rare event, even given the million-plus retinal cells, each of which acts as a potential target for the genetic hit. Which is why children with retinoblastoma that arises by the somatic route don't usually develop more than one tumor. On the other hand, the child inheriting a damaged RB gene, needs only a single additional genetic hit for tumors to take root. Knudson believed that the latter was more likely to occur, with a number of the million retinoblasts sustaining hits. This explained why these children usually form tumors in both eyes.

Because patients with germline retinoblastoma can transmit the faulty gene to half of their offspring, it's essential to suggest prenatal diagnosis as well as asymptomatic carrier testing. Five percent of children with this disease will sustain other congenital defects such as skeletal abnormalities, heart disease, and—most commonly—mental retardation.

For more information on support groups and treatment, contact Leena Hamu, Children's Cancer Group Operations Center, PO Box 60012, Arcadia, CA 91066-6012; (818) 447-0064; American Cancer Society, 1599 Clifton Road NE, Atlanta, GA 30329-4251; 1 (800) ACS-2345; and Cancer Information Service (a program of the National Cancer Institute), 1 (800) 4-CANCER.

Von Hippel-Lindau Disease

In 1904, Dr. Eugen von Hippel described another type of retinal pathology—an angioma, now recognized as part of a larger syndrome called von Hippel-Lindau disease (VHL). Such angiomas also occur in the central nervous system, described in 1926 by Dr. Arvid Lindau. With VHL, cysts and tumors can also appear in the kidney, scrotal sac, pancreas, liver, and adrenal glands.

Scientists have implicated a flaw on chromosome 3 in the VHL gene that normally codes for the von Hippel-Lindau protein (pVHL). Residing in the cytoplasm, pVHL stops tumors from developing. (Among the general population, researchers have found pVHL abnormalities in 85% of kidney cancer tumors.) How the protein performs this task remains unclear. Researchers do know at least one job assigned to pVHL: turn off genes that carry the blueprints for vascular endothelial growth factor (VEGF). Tumors that arise in VHL families secrete such growth factors, which stimulate blood vessel formation. Unless a cell is oxygen deprived, pVHL would normally shut down the release of these growth factors. But a crippled pVHL cannot staunch their flow. Angiomas, cysts, and tumors can follow.

A highly variable disease, VHL manifests differently depending on the codons at which mutations appear. For example, few kidney cancers appear in families with a mutation at codon 505. They tend to contract more adrenal gland and eye tumors, and a few brain tumors. Scientists have traced the 505 mutation to one "founder" who lived in a small village in the Black Forest region of Germany 250 years ago. Some of the founder's descendants emigrated to the United States around 1720 and settled in Pennsylvania. Two of these families, along with 18 in Germany and one in Switzerland who stemmed from the founder, all carry exactly the same mutation.

A flaw at codon 712 has cropped up in different populations around the world, so no one founder can claim it's origin. Berton Zbar, MD, a leading VHL researcher at the National Cancer Institute, speculates that this "weak spot" in the gene sustains damage at different times in different ways. Kidney, brain, eye, and adrenal tumors tend to predominate in families with a flaw at codon 712.

Scientists have not yet located the mutations for at least 20% of VHL families. To better understand the disease, they need to gather more genetic data on these individuals. In the meantime, experts urge regular cancer screening in patients with a family history of VHL, beginning at age six or even earlier.

For more information, contact the VHL Family Alliance at 171 Clinton Road, Brookline, Massachusetts 02146; (617) 232-5946 or (800) 767-4VHL. You can send a fax to (617) 734-8233 or e-mail to vhl@pipeline.com, or visit the Internet web page at http://neurosurgery.mgh.harvard.edu/vhl-fa.

Wilms' Tumor

Once uniformly lethal, the prognosis for this extremely rare (fewer than 500 cases a year reported in the US) childhood renal tumor has changed dramatically. New surgical techniques, improved postoperative care, a recognition of the sensitivity of the Wilms' tumor to radiation, and active chemotherapy agents have greatly reduced the risk of death. As much as 80% of children with even the most advanced stage of the disease will reach 4-year survival. And when physicians detect Wilms' in its earliest stage, fully 95% of patients survive. Doctors usually diagnose the abdominal mass by 33 months of age when the tumors occur bilaterally; unilateral tumors often go undetected until at least 41 months.

Children with Wilms' tumor often exhibit associated disorders: aniridia (absence of an iris), hemihypertrophy (one side of the face or body enlarged), cryptorchidism (failure of one or both testis to descend), and hypospadias (genital malformation). Thus far, researchers have traced the disease and its varied syndromes to at least two genetic flaws located on chromosome 11.

Work conducted by the National Wilms' Tumor Study Group suggests that some bilateral and multicentric tumors may arise from somatic mutations rather than germline flaws. Constitutional or even tumor-specific mutations of the Wilms' tumor gene (WT1) occur in far fewer cases than researchers expected. And in some cases with a tumor-specific WT1 mutation of one allele, the second allele remains normal. Can environmental exposure sustained by fathers somehow trigger this disease? Research has produced conflicting evidence on the risks posed to offspring of auto mechanics, machinists, welders, workers in hydrocarbon-related industries, and those exposed to excess lead.

Because tumors often recur in the lungs of children with stage I or II disease, and in the abdomen of those with stage III and IV, physicians need to conduct careful and frequent follow-up exams, including such measures as palpating the liver, as well as bone and brain scans.

For more information contact Fred Hutchinson Cancer Research Center, 1124 Columbia Street, Seattle, WA 98104;

(206) 667-4842 or (800) 553-4878; American Cancer Society, 1599 Clifton Road NE, Atlanta, GA 30329-4251; 1 (800) ACS-2345; National Cancer Institute's Cancer Information Service, 1 (800) 4-CANCER.

Thyroid Cancer

Hereditary medullary thyroid cancer can strike children as young as 3 months. To diagnose the disease, for the last 20 years physicians have employed the pentagastrin stimulation test, an expensive, uncomfortable exam that can induce esophageal spasms, coughing and vomiting. So poorly do young patients tolerate this calcitonin-measuring test, reports one physician, that some children have taken to swearing at her. Worse, diagnosis of medullary thyroid cancer by pentagastrin lacks specificity. In some cases, when the serum levels showed as much as 5 times the normal amount of calcitonin, surgeons performed thyroidectomies, only to find they had removed histologically normal glands (false positive; false negative tests also occur, delaying cancer diagnosis). Worst of all, once the test reveals abnormalities, the curative window may have already closed.

Without knowing a patient's genetic status, doctors have to repeat the pentagastrin test yearly up to age 30 in those at risk for the syndrome. Only then can they rule out the possibility that a patient will develop the disease. Better to *predict* the disease with genetic testing—the new "gold standard," says Ruth Decker, MD, a thyroid and endocrine surgeon. Gene testing seems all the more urgent, she says, given the fact that with rare exception the predisposing mutation is nearly 100% penetrant. In a family with a history of medullary thyroid cancer, a patient who tests negative could dispense with pentagastrin forever and stop worrying. The patient who tests positive can undergo prophylactic surgery and feel at ease.

Hereditary medullary thyroid cancer falls into three categories:

> Familial medullary thyroid cancer (FMTC)
> Multiple endocrine neoplasia Type 2A (MEN-2A)
> Multiple endocrine neoplasia Type 2B (MEN-2B)

At what age the disease process begins, and how aggressively it develops varies. Recent studies show that perhaps as many as 30 different germline point mutations in the RET proto-oncogene on chromosome 10 correlate to more than 95% of hereditary cases.

Who should seek RET testing? Dr. Decker offers some guidelines:

- Any patient with medullary thyroid cancer, regardless of his or her family history. Up to 30% of medullary thyroid tumors will fall into one of the three types listed above.
- If your patient tests positive, all first-degree relatives, regardless of age. (Tests indicated as early as age three).
- All patients with pheochromocytoma (an adrenal neoplasm); this disease could signal the first hint of the syndromes and that the patient has also inherited the thyroid cancer.
- First-degree relatives of deceased patients who had medullary thyroid cancer.

The 1,500 people who contract thyroid tumors each year in the US and their families can get more information by contacting The Decker Foundation, 7536 Forsyth Boulevard, Suite 91, St. Louis, MO 63105 (800-432-8087).

CHAPTER 6

"Doctor, Do I Need Genetic Testing?"

"Patients are looking for a definitive result.We can't always give them that."

—June A. Peters, MS, Genetic Counselor
National Institutes of Health

Within the next 30 years, primary care doctors will feed a scrap of their patient's DNA into a desktop "gene-alyzer." After some quick calculations, the machine will compare this DNA to a computerized map with key markers, and produce a profile of risks and dispositions. So predicts Arthur Caplan, PhD, head of the Center for Bioethics at the University of Pennsylvania Medical Center. "We will go to a whole new level of diagnostic testing," he says, the logical extension of such tools as cholesterol screens that doctors now use to manage disease and promote healthy lifestyles.

In part, this vision has already been realized. For years, doctors have used gene testing to make prenatal diagnoses, or to identify carriers of Tay-Sachs or cystic fibrosis, for instance. Only recently have they employed this technology for the more complex adult-onset maladies.

Geneticists often tailor cancer tests to specific genes or mutations prevalent in specific families. (It's important to note that a patient cannot undergo testing in a vacuum; clinicians must involve his or her family as well.) And trained genetic counselors guide patients through the maze of risk analysis while helping families grapple with delicate and highly emotional issues.

So where does that leave the general physician whose patient wants to know whether he inherited the genetic mutation for colon cancer because Uncle Jack died of the disease at age 75? Strictly speaking, *hereditary* cancers are linked to mutations in specific genes that follow certain rules of inheritance; *familial* cancers can occur in families at a higher-than-expected rate due to a genetic predisposition to cancer, or a number of nongenetic factors such as lifestyle, hormones, radiation, and other environmental exposures.

Because one in two American men and one in three American women will contract cancer in his or her lifetime, even several cases of cancer in a family do not necessarily mean the disease is hereditary or familial. They could amount to an unlucky streak of *sporadic* cancers—isolated, random events. (In some cases, sporadic cancers *could* prove genetic.)

Uncle Jack's age worked against him; his DNA repair system had too many miles on it to effectively squelch a budding malignancy. If he had contracted the disease at age 45, your patient perhaps should worry that a mutant family gene induced the disease. Most likely, Uncle Jack contracted a sporadic case of cancer—an event that does not raise risk for other family members. But to make certain, you need to probe further to ferret out additional cancers in the family. To identify the small subset of patients and relatives who truly need genetic testing we'll show you step-by-step how to perform triage by:

• Using a decision tree developed by Drs. Stephen Lemon and Henry Lynch at Creighton University to assess cancer risk.

• Constructing a pedigree to augment family histories, visualize disease patterns, and track new cases of cancer.

• Learning when—and to whom—you need to refer patients.

With these skills you will help avoid drowning genetic services in requests for needless tests. And you can free your patients from unnecessary anxiety and expense.

In this chapter we'll also talk about the genetic test itself and what the results mean whether positive, negative, or inconclusive. Chapter 7 will detail family issues and counseling, an important part of what you are about to read.

Assessing Risk: The Decision Tree (see Figure 1)

Step 1: Family history. It's the most basic technique in a doctor's armamentarium: taking a medical history. But surprisingly, many such histories neglect much mention of the family. When it comes to cancer, you need to gather fundamen-

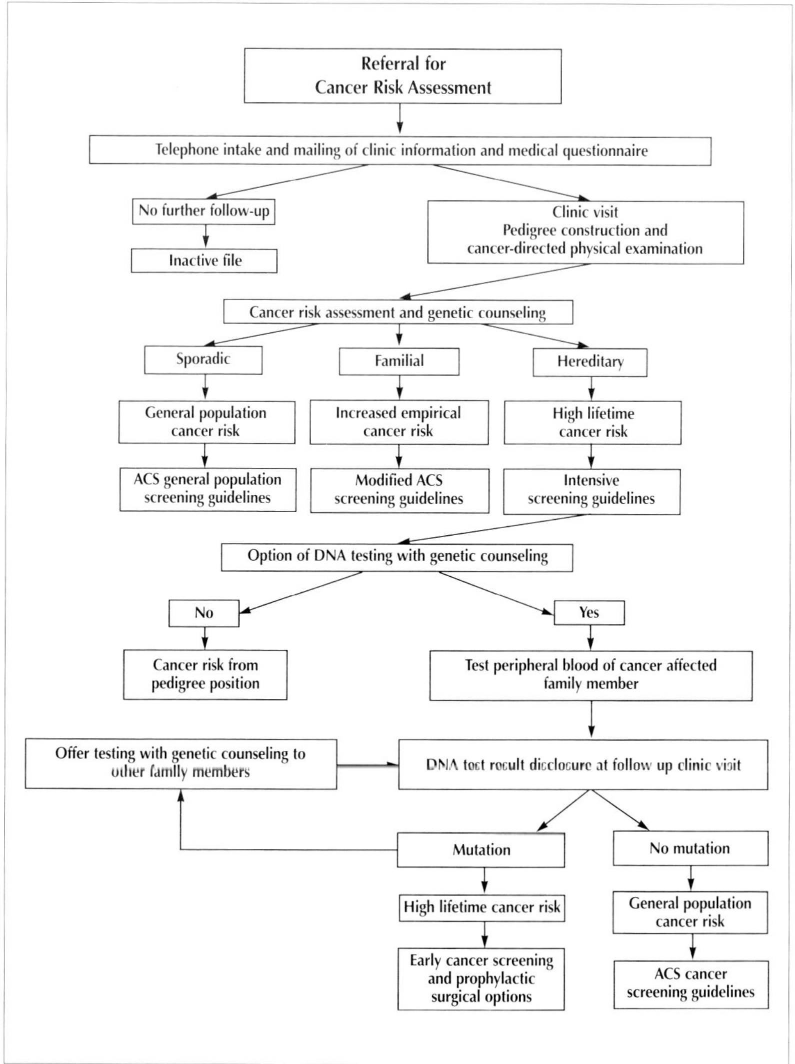

Figure 1: Flow diagram of the Creighton University Hereditary Cancer Prevention Clinic cancer risk assessment and genetic testing process. An extended family tree (pedigree) is constructed showing all cancer occurrences and a cancer-directed physical examination is performed. A cancer risk assessment is made based on this information and communicated to the patient with genetic counseling and appropriate cancer screening guidelines. In those patients diagnosed with a hereditary cancer syndrome associated with an identified gene, the option of DNA testing/counseling is offered both to the patient and to first- and second-degree family members.
ACS = American Cancer Society   DNA = deoxyribonucleic acid

tal information on both maternal and paternal cases. (A number of doctors make the mistake of not asking about breast or ovarian cancer, for instance, among the father's relatives. These may be female diseases, but the genes can dwell in anyone; Dad, for instance, could turn out to carry the BRCA1 mutation.) Other first-degree relatives to ask about: sisters, brothers and children. You also need to find out whether any second-degree relatives—grandparents, aunts, uncles, nieces, nephews, and grandchildren—have had cancer. Cousins—the third-degree relatives—round out the picture.

On the following pages, we provide a sample questionnaire you can copy and distribute to patients; you may want to ask them to fill it out before or after their visit. In that way they can talk with family members who can help gather the information, preferably covering as much as two or more generations.

Steps 2 and 3: Lower Risk or Higher? Genetic counselors refer to cancer risk as higher or lower than the baseline risk of the average person in the population. An increase in risk may rank as statistically slight, moderate, or high. This all sounds academic to a patient; what concerns him is how he *perceives* his risk. And that varies from person to person. Even a low risk of cancer may feel unacceptably dangerous to some. Perhaps one way to approach a discussion of risk with your patients is to refer to it as "higher" or "lower." This subtle but important distinction offers a less threatening and more general way to describe probability. (You might also use the terms "increased" or "decreased" risk.)

It's important to stress to patients that most cancers are *not* inherited. But as you study the completed questionnaire, watch out for the cardinal features of hereditary cancer that should raise your suspicions of a family at higher risk for hereditary cancer syndromes:

- Cancer in two or more close relatives
- Bilateral cancer in paired organs
- Multiple primary tumors in the same individual
- Earlier-than-usual onset of disease
- Specific constellation of tumors that comprise a known cancer syndrome (see Table 1).

<table>
<tr><td colspan="3" align="center">Family Cancer History</td></tr>
<tr>
<td>Your name:</td>
<td colspan="2">Did a doctor ever say that you had cancer?   Yes* / No</td>
</tr>
<tr><td colspan="3">

*If you answered yes, please answer the following five questions:

1. Original location(s) of cancer (colon, breast, lung, etc.): _____________

2. Number of tumors: ______   3. Date of cancer diagnosis: ______

4. Your age at time of diagnosis: ______   5. Did you ever smoke? Yes / No

</td></tr>
<tr>
<td>Your mother's name:</td>
<td>Dates (estimate if unknown)   Birth ______   Death ______</td>
<td>Cause of death:</td>
</tr>
<tr><td colspan="3">

Did she ever have cancer?   Yes* / No

*If yes, please answer the following five questions:

1. Original location(s) of cancer (colon, breast, lung, etc.): ______

2. Number of tumors: ______   3. Date of cancer diagnosis: ______

4. Her age at time of diagnosis: ______   5. Did she ever smoke? Yes / No

</td></tr>
<tr>
<td>Your father's name:</td>
<td>Dates (estimate if unknown)   Birth ______   Death ______</td>
<td>Cause of death:</td>
</tr>
<tr><td colspan="3">

Did he ever have cancer?   Yes* / No

*If yes, please answer the following five questions:

1. Original location(s) of cancer (colon, prostate, lung, etc.): ____________

2. Number of tumors: ______   3. Date of cancer diagnosis: ______

4. His age at time of diagnosis: ______   5. Did he ever smoke? Yes / No

</td></tr>
</table>

Family Cancer History			
Your brother's and/or sister's names	Dates (estimate if unknown) Birth Death	Cause of death	Ever had cancer?
1. _______________	_____ / _____	_______________	Yes / No
2. _______________	_____ / _____	_______________	Yes / No
3. _______________	_____ / _____	_______________	Yes / No
4. _______________	_____ / _____	_______________	Yes / No
Your children's names			
1. _______________	_____ / _____	_______________	Yes / No
2. _______________	_____ / _____	_______________	Yes / No
3. _______________	_____ / _____	_______________	Yes / No
4. _______________	_____ / _____	_______________	Yes / No
Your maternal grandmother's name _______________	_____ / _____	_______________	Yes / No
Your maternal grandfather's name _______________	_____ / _____	_______________	Yes / No
Your paternal grandmother's name _______________	_____ / _____	_______________	Yes / No
Your paternal grandfather's name _______________	_____ / _____ Birth Death	_______________	Yes / No

Family Cancer History				
Locations of cancer	Number of primary tumors	Date of cancer diagnosis	Age at time of diagnosis	Ever smoked?
_____________	_____	_____	_____	Yes / No
_____________	_____	_____	_____	Yes / No
_____________	_____	_____	_____	Yes / No
_____________	_____	_____	_____	Yes / No
_____________	_____	_____	_____	Yes / No
_____________	_____	_____	_____	Yes / No
_____________	_____	_____	_____	Yes / No
_____________	_____	_____	_____	Yes / No
_____________	_____	_____	_____	Yes / No
_____________	_____	_____	_____	Yes / No
_____________	_____	_____	_____	Yes / No
_____________	_____	_____	_____	Yes / No

Family Cancer History

Maternal cousins	Dates (estimate if unknown) Birth / Death	Cause of death	Ever had cancer?
1. _____________	_____ / _____	_____________	Yes / No
2. _____________	_____ / _____	_____________	Yes / No
3. _____________	_____ / _____	_____________	Yes / No
4. _____________	_____ / _____	_____________	Yes / No
5. _____________	_____ / _____	_____________	Yes / No
Paternal cousins			
1. _____________	_____ / _____	_____________	Yes / No
2. _____________	_____ / _____	_____________	Yes / No
3. _____________	_____ / _____	_____________	Yes / No
4. _____________	_____ / _____	_____________	Yes / No
5. _____________	_____ _____	_____________	Yes / No
Grandchildren			
1. _____________	_____ / _____	_____________	Yes / No
2. _____________	_____ / _____	_____________	Yes / No
3. _____________	_____ / _____	_____________	Yes / No
4. _____________	_____ / _____	_____________	Yes / No
5. _____________	_____ / _____	_____________	Yes / No
6. _____________	_____ / _____	_____________	Yes / No
7. _____________	_____ / _____	_____________	Yes / No

Family Cancer History				
Locations of cancer	Number of primary tumors	Date of cancer diagnosis	Age at time of diagnosis	Ever smoked?
————————	————	————	————	Yes / No
————————	————	————	————	Yes / No
————————	————	————	————	Yes / No
————————	————	————	————	Yes / No
————————	————	————	————	Yes / No
————————	————	————	————	Yes / No
————————	————	————	————	Yes / No
————————	————	————	————	Yes / No
————————	————	————	————	Yes / No
————————	————	————	————	Yes / No
————————	————	————	————	Yes / No
————————	————	————	————	Yes / No
————————	————	————	————	Yes / No
————————	————	————	————	Yes / No
————————	————	————	————	Yes / No
————————	————	————	————	Yes / No

Family Cancer History			
Mother's brothers and sisters	**Dates (estimate if unknown)** Birth Death	**Cause of death**	**Ever had cancer?**
1. ______________	______ / ______	______________	Yes / No
2. ______________	______ / ______	______________	Yes / No
3. ______________	______ / ______	______________	Yes / No
4. ______________	______ / ______	______________	Yes / No
Father's brothers and sisters			
1. ______________	______ / ______	______________	Yes / No
2. ______________	______ / ______	______________	Yes / No
3. ______________	______ / ______	______________	Yes / No
4. ______________	______ / ______	______________	Yes / No
Nieces and nephews			
1. ______________	______ / ______	______________	Yes / No
2. ______________	______ / ______	______________	Yes / No
3. ______________	______ / ______	______________	Yes / No
4. ______________	______ / ______	______________	Yes / No
5. ______________	______ / ______	______________	Yes / No
6. ______________	______ / ______	______________	Yes / No
7. ______________	______ / ______	______________	Yes / No
8. ______________	______ / ______	______________	Yes / No
9. ______________	______ / ______	______________	Yes / No

Family Cancer History				
Locations of cancer	Number of primary tumors	Date of cancer diagnosis	Age at time of diagnosis	Ever smoked?
______________________	______	______	______	Yes / No
______________________	______	______	______	Yes / No
______________________	______	______	______	Yes / No
______________________	______	______	______	Yes / No
______________________	______	______	______	Yes / No
______________________	______	______	______	Yes / No
______________________	______	______	______	Yes / No
______________________	______	______	______	Yes / No
______________________	______	______	______	Yes / No
______________________	______	______	______	Yes / No
______________________	______	______	______	Yes / No
______________________	______	______	______	Yes / No
______________________	______	______	______	Yes / No
______________________	______	______	______	Yes / No
______________________	______	______	______	Yes / No

TABLE I

Selected Hereditary Cancer Syndromes

Genetic Condition	Main Cancers	Gene	Location of Mutation	Year Found
Hereditary Retinoblastoma	Retinoblastoma Sarcomas	RBI	13q14	1986
Hereditary Wilms' Tumor	Wilms' Tumor	WTI	11p13	1990
Li-Fraumeni Syndrome	Breast Cancer Sarcomas Brain Tumor	TP53	17p13	1990
Neuro-fibromatosis	Sarcomas Brain Tumor	NFI	17q11	1990
Familial Adenomatous Polyposis	Colon Cancer	APC	5q21	1991
Neuro-fibromatosis 2	Acoustic Neuroma Brain Tumor	NF2	22q12	1993
von Hippel-Lindau Syndrome	Renal Cancer Pheochromocytoma Brain Tumor	VHL	3p25	1993
Multiple Endocrine Neoplasia 2	Pheochromocytoma Medullary Thyroid Cancer	RET	10q11	1993

If you identify a higher risk family, urge them to gather medical documentation, especially pathology reports which contain the most reliable information. Other documents include death certificates, autopsy reports, physician clinic notes, or hospital discharge summaries. Because memories can fail and patients can confuse metastatic and primary tumor sites, for instance, it's essential to confirm cases. Also, some cancer susceptibility genes may predispose a patient to a variety of cancers or other health problems. For example, renal cell carcinoma, pheochromocytoma, retinal angiomas, and cerebellar hemangioblastomas are all associated with von

TABLE I *continued*

Selected Hereditary Cancer Syndromes

Genetic Condition	Main Cancers	Gene	Location of Mutation	Year Found
Tuberous Sclerosis 2	Renal Cancer Brain Tumor	TSC2	16p13	1993
Hereditary Nonpolyposis Colon Cancer	Colon Cancer Cancers of Endometrium, Ovary, Small Bowel, Stomach, Pancreas, Upper Urologic Tract	hMSH2 hMLH1 hPMS1 hPMS2	2p16 3p21 2q32 7p22	1993 1994 1994 1994
Hereditary Melanoma 1	Melanoma	CDKN2	9p21	1994
Hereditary Breast Cancer 1	Breast Cancer Ovarian Cancer	BRCA1	17q21	1994
Ataxia Telangiectasia	Breast Cancer Lymphoma multiple others	ATM	11q22-23	1995
Hereditary Breast Cancer 2	Breast Cancer	BRCA2	13q12-13	1995
Hereditary Melanoma 2	Melanoma Pancreatic Cancer	CDK4	12q13	1996

Hippel-Lindau disease (see Chapter 5).

Referring higher risk patients for counseling and testing. If you do not have a genetics or oncology division at your disposal, you can turn to a number of sources, including the National Society of Genetic Counselors (NSGC) for help. The National Cancer Institute also lists cancer genetics counselors, on their website. You'll find an integrated version of the two lists (NSGC and NCI) in our Appendix 1. You can also search the NCI list on the web: (http://cancernet.nci.nih.gov/wwwprot/genetic/genesrch.html). Most of the counselors are affiliated with research facilities and universities. You can consult with them on ordering specific gene tests. They can recommend commercial laboratories such as OncorMed or Myriad, or university-based labs such as Creighton University's Hereditary Cancer Prevention Clinic or those at Johns Hopkins, to mention a few. The counselors can also coordinate with you your patient's care before and after testing.

Ideally, you can develop a working relationship with these specialists in a team approach to patient care. Even if your patients decide not to go through with testing, speaking with a genetic counselor can go a long way toward easing their fears.

Follow-up

Every family, whether at higher or lower risk for hereditary cancer, can benefit from general cancer education. (If you don't already have information pamphlets you can obtain them by calling the American Cancer Society at 1-800-ACS-2345, or contact the ACS Internet site at http://www.cancer.org). Do emphasize to *all* patients the need for exercise, a low-fat and high-fiber diet, no smoking, reduced alcohol intake, reduced sun exposure, and routine follow-up exams to include:

For women
Regular pap smears
Regular mammograms after age 40 (sooner if relatives have had breast cancer at an early age)
Monthly breast self-exam; yearly clinical exam

For men
Yearly prostate digital exam after age 40
Yearly PSA blood test beginning at age 50

For everyone
Stool test annually after age 50
Flexible sigmoidoscopy every 3-5 years after age 50 or earlier if relatives have had polyps or colon cancer
Digital rectal exam beginning at age 40

Constructing A Pedigree

Many of the hereditary cancer syndromes identified thus far follow autosomal dominant inheritance patterns. At-risk families, therefore, transmit the genes vertically—that is, down the generations. One of the best ways to discern this pattern is with a symbolic picture of the family—a pedigree. Genetics professionals have devised a standard set of symbols for constructing pedigrees (see Figure 2). In this section we'll show you how to build such schematics with two examples from the files of the Mountain States Regional Genetic Services Network. Once you add pedigrees to your patients' medical record, you can easily update the profile over time.

First, a few other elements to look for:

Presence of rare cancers. Chance alone cannot explain clusters of tumors that rarely occur in the general population. For example, Li-Fraumeni syndrome includes cancer of the adrenal gland, a rare tumor. Identifying a family with a group of such cancers points to inheritance.

Cancers in the "wrong" places. Pedigrees that suggest inherited forms of cancer could also include malignancies in unlikely patients: men with breast cancer, for example, or non-smokers with early-onset lung cancer.

The red flags mentioned above in the section on lower and

	Male	Female	Sex Unknown
1. Individual	b. 1925	30 y	4 mo
2. Affected individual			
3. Multiple individuals, number known	5	5	5
4. Deceased individual			
5. Proband	P	P	P

Figure 2: Pedigree Symbols
Adapted from Bennett RL, Steinhous KA, Uhrich SB, et al: Am J Hum Genet 56:745-752, 1995.

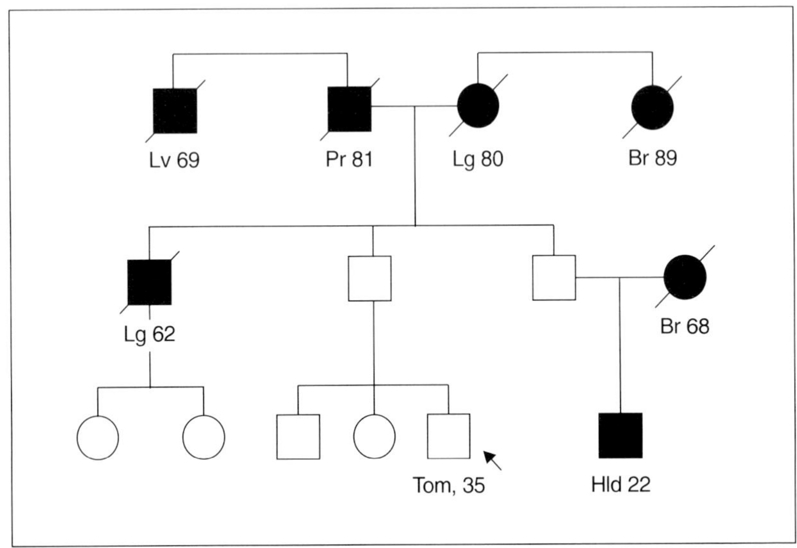

Figure 3: "Everyone in My Family Gets Cancer"—Client concerned with cancer risks due to multiple family members with cancer. See text for discussion of case. Lv = Liver cancer; numeral specifies age at diagnosis; Pr = Prostate cancer; Lg = Lung cancer; Br = Breast cancer; Hld = Hodgkin's lymphoma; Arrow = Client name, current age

higher risks still apply, of course. You may find it easier to recognize them in the "family portrait" —the pedigree.

Case example #1. "Everyone in my family gets cancer." At age 35 Tom felt certain he would develop cancer eventually. While cancer had not struck his mother's side of the family, doctors had diagnosed seven of his paternal relatives with some type of malignancy.

Initially, Tom's story seems to suggest genetic susceptibility to cancer. But when analyzed more closely, the pedigree seems to point away from that. From Figure 3 you can see that Tom has no first degree relatives with cancer. His three affected second-degree relatives, and three affected third-degree relatives come from different sides of the family, which geneticists would consider separately. Note that one of the breast cancer cases occurd in an aunt by marriage (Br 68), not a blood relation.

As we've said, families with inherited forms of cancer include multiple members affected with the same or related types of malignancies. Leaving aside the paternal aunt, Tom's family includes two members with lung cancer, one with breast cancer, one with prostate cancer, one with liver cancer, and one with Hodgkin's lymphoma. Such a combination of cancers does not comprise a known cancer syndrome, and none of these tumors is especially rare.

Note that family members developed tumors at expected ages—that is to say late onset. Tom's cousin contracted Hodgkin's at age 22, normal for that disease, and all other malignancies occurred in people over 60, also common. Cancers of late onset imply sporadic, not hereditary origin.

It turns out that Tom's uncle, grandfather, and great-uncle all smoked cigarettes for many years. And Tom's great-uncle who died of liver cancer also had a history of alcoholism. So you could attribute their cancers, at least in part, to nongenetic environmental factors. Tom, too, confesses to smoking one pack a day.

Conclusion: A hereditary cancer syndrome does not seem to run in this family. But given the history of lung cancer in relatives who smoked, Tom's doctor advised him to quit smoking in order to reduce his risk. (Studies show that cigarette smokers from lung cancer-prone families tend to run a higher risk of contracting the disease than do smokers in the general population who do not have lung cancer in their family.) And because Tom's grandfather contracted prostate cancer, the doctor also recommended that Tom follow standard screening guidelines for that disease.

Case example #2: Two Sides To Every Family.

Paula, age 36, came to her doctor worried about con-

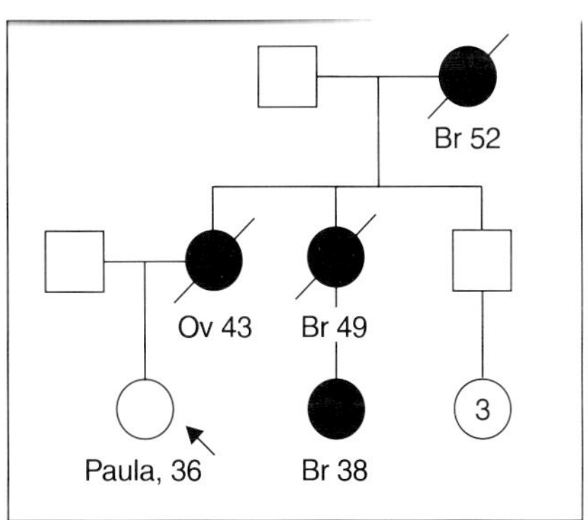

Figure 4: Two Sides to Every Family. Initial pedigree reveals family history of early-onset breast and ovarian cancer. See text for discussion of case. Br = Breast cancer; numeral = age at diagnosis; Ov = Ovarian cancer; 3 = 3 unaffected female siblings; Arrow = Client name, current age.

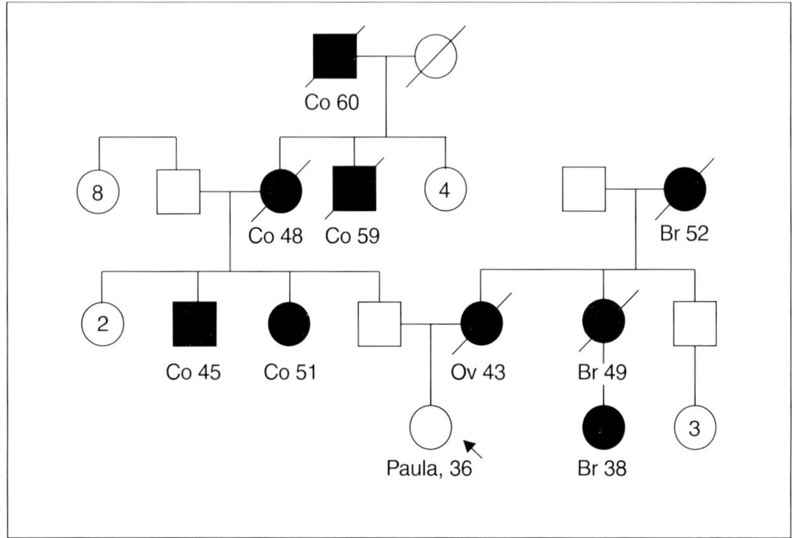

Figure 5: Two sides to every family. Final pedigree reveals maternal relatives with early-onset breast and ovarian cancer and paternal relatives with early-onset colon cancer. See text for discussion of diagnosis. Age at diagnosis: Co - Colon cancer; Br = Breast cancer; Ov = Ovarian cancer; 2 = Number of unaffected female siblings; Arrow = Client name, current Age.

tracting breast and ovarian cancer. She had good reason: her mother had ovarian cancer; her maternal grandmother, maternal aunt, and the aunt's daughter had each developed breast cancer. All these women were diagnosed between the ages of 38 and 52. Paula's doctor drew her pedigree (see Figure 4); it seemed likely that a genetic test could reveal a faulty BRCA1 gene in the family.

But there was more. So focused was she on breast and ovarian cancer, Paula neglected to mention, nor was she asked, about other cancers in the family. And here is where the pedigree picture darkens even further. Five of Paula's paternal relatives in three generations had developed early-onset colon cancer (see Figure 5), putting her at a higher risk for inheriting this disease as well.

Moral of the story: even if a patient presents with questions about a specific disease, it may take more than one go-round to complete the picture. Paula expressed much surprise and distress when she learned of her risk for developing colon cancer. But

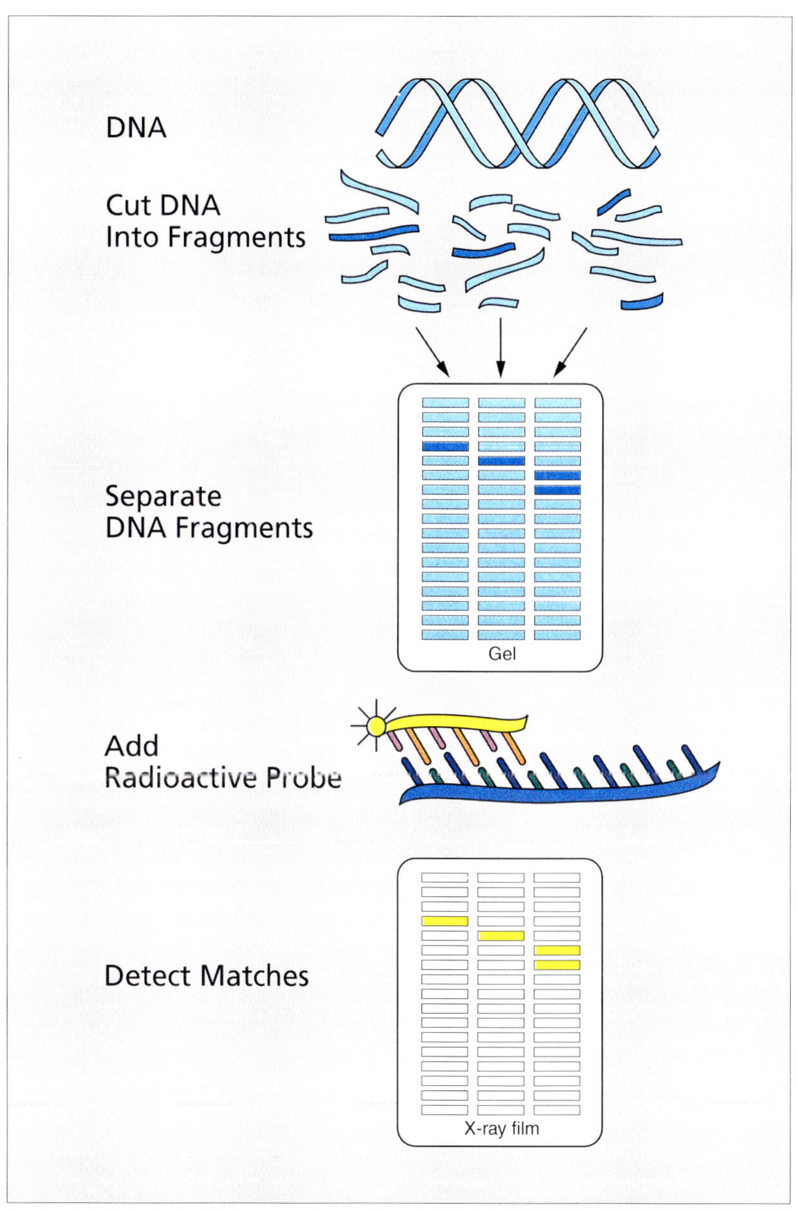

Figure 6: To find a gene mutation in a sample of DNA, scientists use a DNA probe—a length of single-stranded DNA that matches part of the gene and is linked to a radioactive atom. The single-stranded probe seeks and binds to the gene. Radioactive signals from the probe are then made visible on x-ray film, showing where the probe and gene matched.

now she knows information vital to making health care decisions.

As you will see in the following chapters, patients need a careful discussion of test results, with counseling before and after testing to weigh their fears, anxieties, the potential for family strife, and discrimination in hiring and insurance. They need information on the natural history of their family's cancer syndrome, plus appropriate screening and management. Experts strongly advise against submitting blood for testing to any laboratory that does not also provide psychological support.

The Genetic Tests Available

More than 1,500 years ago, Talmudic scholars described a genetic test performed by rabbis. If a male child bled heavily after circumcision, the rabbis exempted from this ancient ritual any brothers born later. They also excused any sons born to the sisters of women whose male children had bled profusely. But if the father of one of these children remarried, the rabbis reinstated the ceremony. Even in that time, long before the era of molecular biology, they knew that hemophilia runs in families from mothers to sons. Now we call that pattern "X-linked recessive."

Today's predictive gene tests can identify the person at risk of contracting hereditary cancer before symptoms ever appear. To burrow into a patient's DNA and emerge with a cancer gene, researchers perform a linkage analysis, looking for genetic markers consistently inherited by those with the disease (see Chapter 2). They then launch a gene probe—a piece of single-stranded DNA that matches parts of the known gene. This probe seeks and binds to complementary bases in the gene. When tagged with a radioactive atom, the probe acts as a lighted beacon to mark the gene's location (Figure 6). Once geneticists find the neighborhood in which to search, they can find the precise gene mutation.

Among the cancer genetic tests now available:

Retinoblastoma and Wilms' tumor (see Chapter 5).

Li-Fraumeni. Those in rare cancer-prone families can be tested in commercial or academic laboratories or can enter research studies.

Familial adenomatous polyposis (see Chapter 4). Researchers have now developed a test for the damaged gene that triggers the tendency to form hundreds of colon polyps, some of which can turn cancerous unless removed. However, doctors can diagnose the condition without the gene test.

Hereditary nonpolyposis colon cancer (Chapter 4). As many as 1 million Americans may carry a mutation in one of the genes that cause perhaps as much as 60% of all inherited colon cancers. HNPCC mutations have been linked to cancers of the colon, endometrium, stomach, ovary, small intestine, kidney, and ureter. Scientists now offer gene tests to families at increased risk—those with three or more affected members (at least one before age 50), over two or more generations.

Breast and ovarian cancer (see Chapter 3). Aside from testing in a number of clinical settings, at least one commercial lab has advertised directly to patients, urging them to seek testing for BRCA1 and BRCA2. This approach is not prudent. One should receive genetic counseling before testing and at time of disclosure. We should only test when clearly indicated. While the picture of risk is changing, the breast cancer risk to patients with BRCA1 or BRCA2 germline mutations may be as high as 85% over their lifetime. However, this risk may vary in any given family with these germline mutations. Nevertheless, the majority of women carrying BRCA1 or BRCA2 germline mutations and who are members of well-defined hereditary cancer prone families will develop one or more cancers of the breast and/or ovary during their lifetime. Exact risk figures should be tailored to age, to personal history of cancer, to known family history in a given case and to the nature and frequency of the particular mutation identified. Men carrying mutations may also be at risk for development of cancers, particulary of the prostate and colon. However, the full cancer spectrum of BRCA1 and BRCA2 germline mutations awaits further retrospective and prospective investigation.

Positive, negative, inconclusive

When you order a cholesterol test for a patient you get a straightforward answer from the lab: you know exactly how many milligrams per deciliter exist in the blood, the ratio of HDL to LDL, the level of triglycerides. But in the world of genetic testing for cancer, answers don't shake out quite so clearly. "A lot of people don't realize the level of uncertainty involved," says June Peters, a genetic counselor with the National Center for Human Genome Research.

If the test comes back positive, it's still not clear when or if that patient will contract cancer. What the patient does know is that he or she can pass the faulty gene to their children.

If the test comes back negative, that doesn't mean the patient has received some special cancer dispensation; he still retains the same risk as the rest of the population. And the negative result pertains *only* to the particular mutation targeted—presumably the one causing cancer in that family. If the cause is unknown and the patient tests negative, he could still carry a higher risk for some other gene.

Then there is the inconclusive result: In some cases, it's not clear what, if anything, the altered nucleotides mean. Researchers would need to find and test big families with this same small change in order to know.

How Useful Are the Tests?

Given the uncertainties, your patients may well ask: Of what use are these tests? For people in higher risk families with a known mutation in a cancer susceptibility gene, a negative test can provide a sense of relief. Instead of living on tenterhooks, they can embrace their hopes and dreams. The results may also allow them to curtail their number of burdensome checkups and tests such as colonoscopy. Conversely, a positive test can help people focus on making decisions about their future. Patients may feel empowered knowing they increase their odds of beating cancer if they catch it early through screening and healthful lifestyle. Some may even choose a preemptive strike with prophylactic surgery.

Making the decision to submit to gene testing can mean choosing a path fraught with emotional peril. In Chapter 7 you'll hear the extraordinary story of a family haunted by cancer dozens of times, working with researchers to track nearly 900 relatives. It's a cautionary tale of how breaking open old fears created painful new wounds. But it's also a tale of strength and resolve.

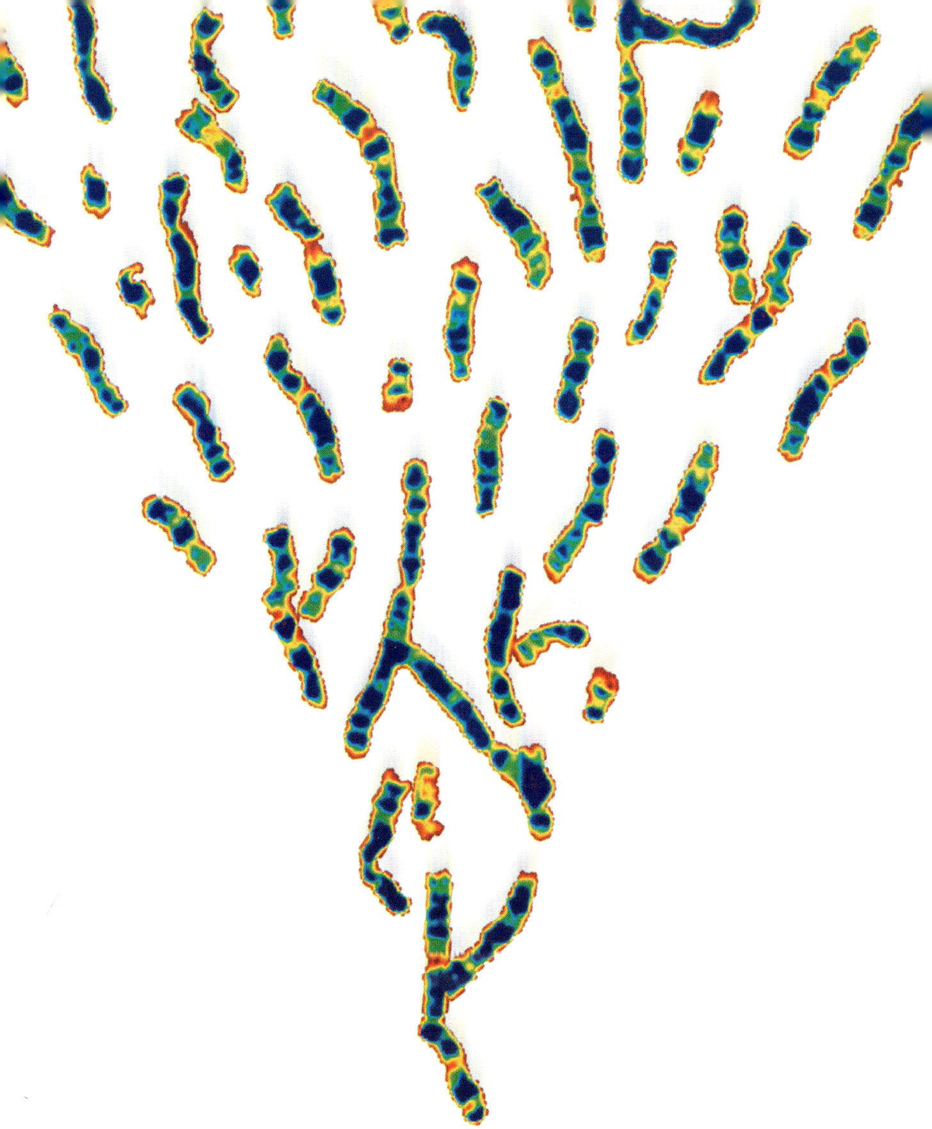

A new force in gene therapy

Creating a new and expanded vision in
gene therapy and cancer research.

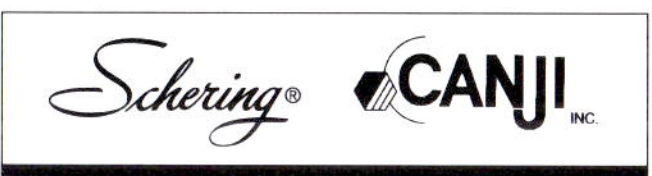

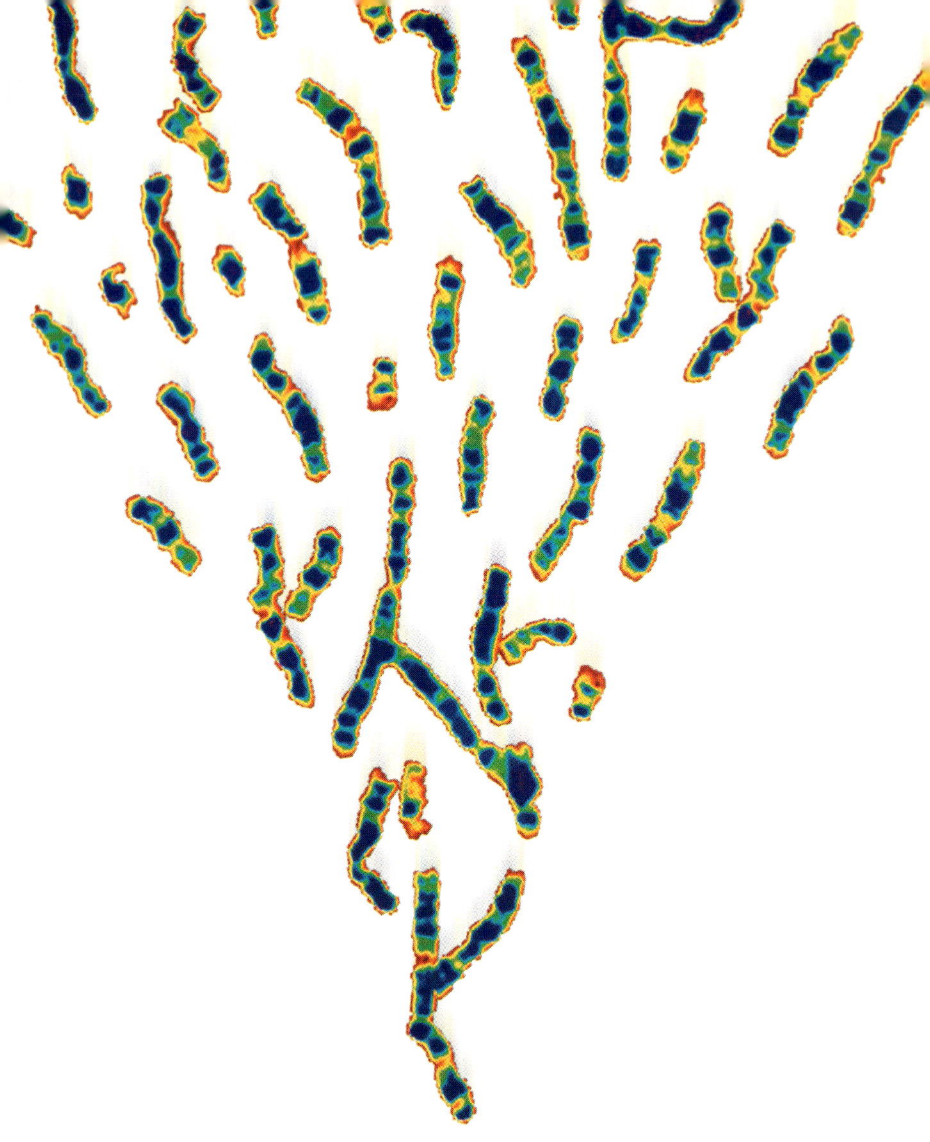

A new force in gene therapy

Creating a new and expanded vision in
gene therapy and cancer research.

CHAPTER 7

Facing Family Issues

"The patient is the family."

—*Genetic counselors' adage*

ounseling patients on whether they should seek genetic testing means taking time to listen. And often, what you will hear is the sound of family secrets breaking loose: buried anger or guilt when one sibling lives cancer-free while another struggles with disease; feelings of shame and blame; conflicts when one family member wants to uncover information that another feels is best left untouched.

In this chapter we focus on family dynamics and the profound adjustments needed when new genetic information comes to light. There's no better way to illustrate this than with the real-life story of Phyllis Hall, told in her own words. Hereditary breast and ovarian cancer struck Hall's family dozens of times.* After generations of illness and death and worry, in 1992 the family could finally find some answers in a genetic test for BRCA1 mutations. But behind every answer lay a new question and a new anxiety.

In Hall's story you will see first-hand the range of emotions and conflicts that can bubble up when people face genetic testing. And you'll hear suggestions culled from a variety of experts on how to help your patients and their families deal with these struggles pre- and post-testing.

A Cancer Legacy

This story begins in rural Minnesota in the 1800s where an immigrant family settles in America and produces 14 children

---

* By studying this extraordinary family, scientists at Creighton University clinched the link between these two cancers. For more on that, see Chapter 3.

to help work the farm. A strong Catholic clan, they pass on their religious values. Four of the children will also pass on to their descendants a mutant BRCA1 gene.

Phyllis Hall, a 49-year-old oncology nurse, can trace her 900-member pedigree back to her great-grandmother, one of 14 siblings, who died of breast cancer in her 40s. As long as Hall can remember, cancer has dogged her family:

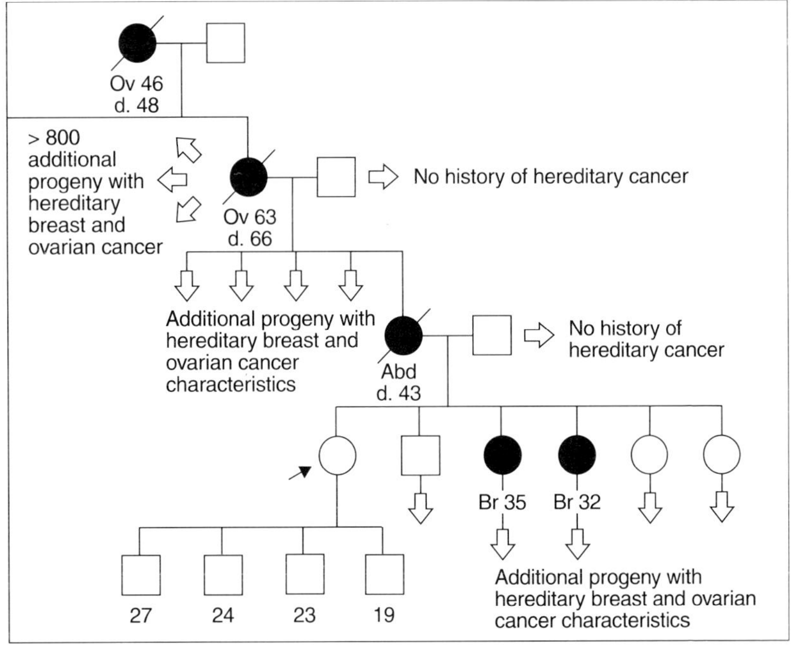

Figure 1: Phyllis Hall's family pedigree

"My first recollection was when I was 5 years old and I went to a wake for my great-great-Aunt Sadie. I remember where the casket lay in the house, the flowers, the music. I remember sprinkling holy water on Aunt Sadie and kneeling with my mother to say a prayer. After that, we experienced one diagnosis and death after another. In 1966, when I was 16, my grandmother was diagnosed with ovarian cancer and died two years later. In 1970 my 43-year-old mother was diagnosed with gastric cancer and died 11 months later. I was 23 years old at the time, married with one child. My brother was 21, and my sisters were 16, 13, 10 and 7. Of Mom's seven sisters, five have been diagnosed with either breast or ovarian cancer and only one is a long-term survivor.

"Early in our marriage my husband and I made very clear life choices based on the family cancer history. He and I decided not to have children after we turned 30. I made a private bargain with God that if he let me see my children graduate from high school I'd be ready to accept death if that was what he intended for me.

"In 1980 my 43-year-old Aunt Helen was diagnosed with a second breast cancer. The doctors at Mayo Clinic recommended that women in our family over age 30 consider prophylactic mastectomy, and prophylactic oophorectomy when they completed childbearing. Two of my aunts, age 38 and 40, had the surgery almost immediately. I struggled with the decision for a year before I had a bilateral mastectomy. A year after that Aunt Helen died.

"My sisters had much more difficulty deciding on preventive surgery. They were 7 to 16 years younger than I. At age 32, my sister Taunia was diagnosed with breast cancer. Seven months later my sister Tammy received the same diagnosis; she was 35. And my first cousin Paula was then diagnosed at age 30. (Note that Hall has 47 first cousins on her mother's side alone!)

"By this time we were documenting our family history and I learned that many of the cancers identified as stomach and 'female cancers' were actually ovarian tumors. So I chose to have oophorectomy. At the same time my two youngest sisters, age 25 and 28 had prophylactic mastectomies. I know that these surgeries are controversial. But a family like ours doesn't have many options. In the past the women in our family have not lived long after their cancer diagnoses. Now, for the first time our generation is seeing survivors."

"Making the decision to have prophylactic surgery requires that you come to terms with your sexuality. I am so fortunate because my husband's loving support has helped me separate my sexuality from body parts. Unfortunately, others in my family have not enjoyed that kind of support. One of my sister's marriage ended in divorce. Her husband increased her stress and confusion. He was an obstacle to her survival. She underwent prophylactic oophorectomy and he could not accept the need for her to undergo prophylactic mastectomy as well. She delayed the breast surgery. Six months after doctors removed her ovaries she was diagnosed with breast cancer. Eighteen months after that her breast cancer recurred. But since her divorce she relocated, started a wonderful new job, and created a stable life for her children. She relies on family and friends for emotional support. She is a 7-year survivor.

The Testing Dilemma

"When Dr. Henry Lynch and his team at Creighton University gave us the chance to take a test for our carrier status, my siblings and I never considered not getting the results. It was information we needed for ourselves and our children. We operated on the premise that knowledge is power, and armed with knowledge we could make the best individual decisions possible.

"Many family members who took part in the linkage analysis studies chose not to receive their results. They could not face the finality of that information. One of my aunts felt that because she had not been diagnosed with breast or ovarian cancer by the time she was 50, then she didn't have the mutation. She failed to understand the concepts of gene penetrance and lifetime risk. Now that her two sons are old enough to marry, she has decided to learn her BRCA1 status for their benefit.

"My sisters and I always assumed that we carried the gene; it was a fact of life. My brother, like many males in the family, thought he didn't. Although the counselors explained autosomal dominance to us several times, the men continued to believe this is a female problem.

"I was the first to receive the information that I did not have the mutation. As soon as the news registered in my brain I realized that if I didn't have it, most likely one of my other siblings did. My heart fell to my feet. When they told my 29-year-old sister with two small children that she had the mutation I felt like I'd been stabbed. Before my mother died I promised her I would take care of my sisters. I felt like I had failed. Two of my sisters had already been diagnosed with breast cancer and now I find out that another has the BRCA1 mutation. How could I feel happy about my carrier status when one of my siblings was affected?

"That night my husband and I sat up the whole night talking. Our lives had changed in a split second with this new information. We talked about things we had never discussed in 20 years of marriage: grandchildren, growing old together, retirement. I had never allowed myself to envision any of that."

A Counselor in the Family

"Every day after my family learned of our carrier status, I called my sister who has the mutation to let her express her feelings, so she could let out her anger, pain, and tears. First she mourned, and then she began to take charge of her life. She made consultation appointments with several physicians. It was very hard for the doctors to handle her approach. They thought she was coming in to be examined, but she and her husband were there to interview the doctors. She wanted to find a physician they felt comfortable with, one who under- stood the implications of her carrier status. She wanted a doctor they could work with to design a surveillance and prevention program.

"I felt embarrassed by my survivor's guilt and so didn't discuss it with anyone. I thought there was something wrong with me. I lived so long believing I would die from cancer I didn't know how to think differently. My job raising children was almost over and I was ready to deal with cancer. Now I had to re-focus my life."

Family Rifts

"Never once have I or my youngest sister, who also tested negative, ever regretted our prophylactic surgeries. We both feel we made the best decisions possible with the information available to us at the time. In a close family like ours it's difficult for some to respect the rights of others to make their own decisions. Some relatives have used pressure to change another's mind about preventive surgery or carrier testing.

"For instance, my first cousin Bridgett's older sister was diagnosed with breast cancer at age 30. Their mother died from ovarian cancer at age 49. Bridgett herself carries the mutated BRCA1 gene. She and I have talked a number of times about her decision not to have prophylactic surgery. I have tried to support Bridgett in this decision. For her it's the best choice regardless of what others think. Her siblings keep trying to persuade her to have the surgery. And they express frustration with my approach—what genetic counselors refer to as acting in a 'nondirective' way.

"I sat with my aunt and uncle the day their daughter Brenda had a bilateral mastectomy for breast cancer and prophylactic hysterectomy and oophorectomy. Brenda's father, a BRCA1 carrier, always thought this was a female problem. But the day of the surgery I could see his unbelievably intense pain. He felt so guilty for passing this genetic mutation to his daughter. She has told him many times that she does not hold him responsible, that she isn't angry with him, that she loves him and is glad he brought her into the world. But he still has a very difficult time dealing with his carrier status. And he can't talk with anyone about his feelings. Sometimes he even tells people he doesn't have the mutated gene.

"The first few weeks after her surgery, Brenda said she felt angry with her sister. They had been very close, had shared everything and done everything together. Now Brenda had to face cancer alone; she carried the gene and her sister didn't. It wasn't fair. But with the help and support of their mother and other cousins, these two sisters now feel as close as ever. They were able to get beyond the anger and pain."

Please Tell Me Again

"Frequently people in hereditary cancer families need to hear an explanation of genetic information more than once. When one of my cousins was diagnosed with premenopausal breast cancer, she told other cousins it was a case of sporadic cancer, not due to the BRCA1 gene. The news spread through our family like wildfire and many relatives called me to verify this information. I referred them back to Creighton University. "When Dr. Lynch next visited Minnesota he spoke with this cousin and her parents to explain her diagnosis again.

Sometimes a new diagnosis or death can stir up anxiety,

stress and confusion. It means that people have to mourn their losses again before they can move forward. In the literature they call it chronic sorrow. I call it recurring sorrow or grief. Additional counseling and support groups can help."

A Family's Strength

"Although we have been plagued by diagnoses at young ages, shortened life expectancies, and children growing up without the guidance of their mothers, you will not see despair in my family. We take a pragmatic approach, believing that what you do with your life is more important than how long you live. Our legacy of cancer has brought us together. We developed support systems within the family. We have learned to reach out to each other in very caring ways."

First Listen...

In Shakespeare's *King Henry IV, Part II*, Falstaff complains, "It is the disease of not listening, the malady of not marking, that I am troubled withal." In a way, the Bard presaged this notion: The best medicine you can offer your patients before and after genetic testing is to listen to them. For some patients these counseling sessions offer the first chance to talk about a painful family history and the death of many loved ones. It may take more than one session to work through their grief before patients can focus on what you discuss about testing, what it could mean to them, and what the results could imply for medical care. You and your staff need to help your patients gently peel away the layers of sadness, anxiety, or fear that can make it difficult for them to absorb "the facts of the case."

Don't be surprised if patients see-saw between wanting testing and rejecting it, between wanting to know the results and shunning them. Only when you have explored all the issues together can this "back-and-forth" level out and the patient feel firmly about his or her choice. In a few cases, genetic testing can cause such acute distress, you may have to refer your patient for psychiatric help. Panic, severe depression, and suicidal thoughts all warrant intervention.

...Then Talk

When you feel your patient is ready to talk about the pros and cons of seeking gene testing, try the following steps. This strategy is based on a number of sources, including research reported by Lois J. Loescher, MS, RN, of the University of Arizona Cancer Center in Tucson, (*Oncology Nursing Forum* 22(suppl 2), 1995) as well as recommendations of psychologists, genetic counselors, bioethicists, and the NIH Task Force on Genetic Testing:

- Find out how much your patient knows about cancer and cancer risk.
- Identify and correct misconceptions.
- Pay attention to emotional reactions, such as fear, that block comprehension.
- Stay sensitive to cultural or religious differences that affect a patient's point of view.
- Recognize that risk perception differs from one person to the next.
- Point out the difference between risk of disease and risk of death.
- Acknowledge that science cannot answer many questions concerning genetics and cancer.
- Repeat the information in varied ways to help your patient better understand. Be prepared to re-visit the discussion at a later date if necessary.
- Don't overload patients with too much information at one time.
- Stress that testing is voluntary and support whatever decision your patient reaches.
- Refrain from making your own preferences known.
- Disclose any conflict of interest you may have in referring patients for testing; for example, if you have a financial stake in a clinical laboratory, or would benefit from the referral.
- Encourage parents, in most cases, *not* to test their children. For adult-onset cancers, knowing a child's genetic status will not affect the course of the disease or its treatment and could affect how parents treat their children, by being overprotective, for instance. Medical ethicists point out that testing a child who cannot consent or refuse robs them of their rights.

TABLE I.

Some Professional Education Resources on Cancer Genetics

Organization	Program
Fox Chase Cancer Center 215-728-2892	Familial Cancer Risk Counseling: An Educational Program for Nurses
University of Iowa 319-335-7608	Genetics and Nursing, Basic Principles Practice
Creighton University Hereditary Cancer Institute 402-280-2941	Hereditary Cancer Syndrome Diagnosis, Genetic Counseling, Surveillance and Management Recommendations

Adapted from The Information Sources: Cancer Genetics and Genetic Testing. Cancer Practice, November/December 1996, Volume 4, No. 6.

When a child reaches maturity, can weigh the options and handle the results, then he or she can decide what to do.

• Schedule follow-up sessions post-testing to discuss the results and emotional fall-out.

• Do not inform other family members of test results without the expressed written permission of the person tested, except in extreme circumstances—that is, if failing to relay the information would cause irreversible or fatal harm.

For more information on counseling training, see Table 1 above.

CHAPTER 8

Discrimination and Privacy

"For the clinical oncologist, the primary care provider, the person with cancer and those at risk for cancer, these are confusing times."

—*Karen Rothenberg, JD, MPA*
Director, Law and Healthcare Program
University of Maryland School of Law

Whenever Maria Burke* met with a doctor, she dutifully answered questions about her medical history—in particular, the many relatives struck by breast cancer in her family: great grandmother, grandmother, mother, maternal aunt.

"When I first heard about genetic testing I was so excited," says Maria. "I thought it would solve a lot of issues I was dealing with. But I wish I had never talked about my family history because I now know it can be used against me. And I do not want a genetic test done until I can control the release of that information as well. I'm amazed that this test, this wonderful technology, is such a two-edged sword. It can actually put you at a bigger risk emotionally and financially than if you had never taken it."

Maria says she has "no doubt the breast cancer gene mutation runs in my family. But if all I can do about it is be aggressive about regular checkups and mammograms—well, I do that anyway. So I don't want to take the test and therefore take the risk of losing my job or my insurance."

Here is a patient who actually wishes she had kept important medical information from her doctor. She knows the laws do not protect her fully, so she prefers playing dice with her health rather than risk losing her livelihood. And she turned away a high-tech medical test because she knows that even though the test may predict disease, her doctors cannot always

---

* Not her real name

prevent or cure the disease.

As your patients consider genetic testing, you will want to discuss with them the issues we touch on in this chapter.

Fears Perceived and Realized

Maria's story echoes across the country. Recently, when researchers at Georgetown University studied more than 300 members of genetics support groups, they heard an earful of complaints about discrimination. Nearly half the respondents asked about genetic diseases on health insurance applications said they were denied coverage. Eighty-three percent said they would not want their insurers to know if they were tested and found to be at high risk for a genetic disorder. Fear of discrimination forced 9% of the subjects to refuse testing and 18% from revealing test results to insurers.

On-the-job concerns were similar: 87% said they would not want their employers to know if they were tested and found at high risk for a genetic disorder. Thirteen percent said they or another family member had been denied a job or fired because of a genetic condition.

Genes in the Workplace

When it comes to access to genetic information in medical records, employers feel entitled to range through patients' private files. Because for them, even the hint of a disease-to-come rings alarm bells in the accounting department: this person could turn into an expensive burden. For some employers, an "at-risk" finding constitutes a pre-existing condition. Never mind the fact that the employee has yet to show symptoms—and may never even contract the disease.

So what protects an employee from bias based on genetic heritage? According to an analysis by Karen Rothenberg of the University of Maryland Law and Healthcare Program, only 11 states address, to varying degrees, genetic findings and the workplace:

Florida	Iowa	Wisconsin
Louisiana	New Hampshire	Oregon
New Jersey	New York	Rhode Island
North Carolina	Oklahoma (a study commission only)	

In the 1970s North Carolina and Florida moved to protect African Americans from bias in hiring and insurance practices because of sickle cell test results. Neither of these states has subsequently passed laws that would expand protections to other disorders.

In 1992 Iowa lawmakers, for instance, forbade employers from requiring a genetic test as a condition of employment. Rothenberg points out the problem with this and most of the other genes-in-the-workplace laws: they focus too narrowly on the genetic *test* rather than more broadly on genetic *information*. This means that patients (as well as their family members to whom the information also applies) still run a risk of discrimination. Under these laws, employers could demand— and get—a general medical release that contains family history data, medical exam or other records. Even without a genetic test, these types of records contain enough genetic information to point to people at risk for cancer, for example, and thus could lead to bias in hiring.

In order to fight genetic discrimination, employees can seek protection under the Americans with Disabilities Act (ADA). The Equal Employment Opportunity Commission issued guidelines saying that the ADA protects from bias those with increased susceptibility to cancer as predicted by positive gene test results. (However, when people use this act as a shield, they must break the seal on their privacy by showing they have a gene defect.)

Health Insurance Discrimination

By 1991, says Rothenberg, a new crop of state laws dealing with health insurance issues began to evolve when Wisconsin lawmakers tried to combine protection against insurance discrimination with protection against privacy violations. They passed a law that prohibited health insurers from:
• requiring or requesting an individual or a member of his family to submit to a genetic test;
• requiring or requesting directly or indirectly the results of a genetic test;
• offering insurance coverage or benefits only on the condition that the applicant take a genetic test;

• using genetic testing results to determine the cost of premiums.

To varying degrees, 13 states have addressed health insurance issues:

Alabama	California	Colorado
Florida	Georgia	Maryland
Minnesota	New Hampshire	North Carolina
Ohio	Oregon (study commission only)	
Virginia	Wisconsin	

A number of other states have legislation pending.

It's worth noting, says Rothenberg, that under Ohio law, if a patient voluntarily submits favorable test results an insurer may consider the data in their decision making.

From the start of the Human Genome Project, scientists at the National Center for Human Genome Research (NCHGR) recognized that gene-finding technologies could spawn a number of complex policy questions. So the NCHGR set aside 5% of its annual research budget to study a number of "ethical, legal, and social implications" (ELSI) of genetic research. In 1995, the ELSI Working Group and the National Action Plan for Breast Cancer made a number of health insurance recommendations, endorsed by the American Cancer Society. Insurance providers, they suggested, should be prohibited from:

• releasing genetic information without the prior written authorization of the individual. Written authorization should be required for each disclosure and include to whom the disclosure would be made;

• using genetic information or an individual's request for genetic services to deny or limit coverage, or establish eligibility, continuation, enrollment, or contribution requirements;

• requesting or requiring collection or disclosure of genetic information;

• establishing different rates or premium payments based on genetic information.

The recommendations stressed that genetic information be defined as "information about genes, gene products, or inherited characteristics that may derive from the individual or a family member."

Federal Health Insurance Protections

Among the provisions of the newly passed Health Insurance Portability and Accountability Act: In group health plans paid for by employers, insurers cannot treat genetic findings as a pre-existing condition in the absence of a diagnosis. If a healthy patient tests positive for a mutation to the BRCA1 gene, for instance, the insurer cannot limit her care if she develops breast cancer in the future.

Under this new federal law, Rothenberg points out, while insurers may not discriminate against an individual, they could still impose a blanket policy not to cover prophylactic mastectomies or oophorectomies, for instance. Or, they may agree to fund mammograms only once every 2 years but not once every 6 months, an increased surveillance plan that some patients could require. They may exclude coverage for a particular condition or procedure, and may impose lifetime caps on benefits.

Something else worth noting: This new federal law does not address whether insurers may request genetic information or require doctors to collect it. And insurers need not obtain authorization before disclosing test results. Some insurers warn that if new laws do limit their access to genetic information, it will undercut their ability to classify risk. That, they say, would force them to raise premiums, placing insurance beyond the reach of many people, especially those who underwrite their own policies. A few insurers even go so far as to predict that as a result of these laws, ultimately the sky will fall on an insolvent industry.

Issues To Think About

"Americans," George Bernard Shaw lamented in 1933, "have no sense of privacy; there is no such thing in the country," he said. Shaw could not have known how much "more true" that statement would ring 60 years later because now, of course, the invasion of our privacy can extend all the way down to our genes. It doesn't get more personal than that.

In your own record keeping, how can you insure your patient's privacy? By writing down your discussions of family history, you may inadvertently jeopardize your patient's health insurance coverage the next time his carrier requests records. Perhaps you want to consider keeping sensitive material such as HIV results, abortion history, and genetic data in special "shadow files." You might also want to consider ways to work with advocacy groups, your state legislature, Congress, and insurance companies to resolve these policy issues.

Experts characterize the current picture as "a patchwork and a mess." There is no guarantee of privacy and no guarantee of confidentiality, even in research records. Says Rothenberg, "that is a real risk. We hope it's not a real harm."

APPENDIX I

Familial Cancer Risk Counseling and Genetic Testing Information

*The following list of cancer genetic counselors was compiled from two sources: One was the National Cancer Institute listing on their website (**http://cancernet.nci.nih.gov/wwwprot/genetic/genesrch.html**). The second was the membership of the National Society of Genetic Counselors (NSGC) Cancer Risk Counseling Special Interest Group. **Members of the NSGC special interest group are designated with an asterisk.* For** further information, you can contact the NCI website at the address above, or write to the NSGC, attention: Ms Bea Leopold, 233 Canterbury Drive, Wallingford, PA 19086-6617; Fax: 610-872-1192. Readers should be aware that all of these counselors may not be trained to counsel patients regarding every kind of genetic cancer, such as Von Hippel-Lindau Disease, etc. Thus in inquiring of any one counselor, readers should ask about his or her particular qualifications.*

Also, please bear in mind that lists such as these are always in a state of flux: people move, phone numbers change, new names are added. Thus, if you fail to reach a particular counselor at the address / phone number listed here, you might check the NCI website as shown above or fax the NSGC office.

Alabama

*Ronald T. Acton, PhD**
University of Alabama
Birmingham
Phone: 1-800-GXY-GENE
or 205 934-2362
Fax: 205 934-4062

Arizona

*Amy Cronister, MS**
Mayo Clinic
Familial Cancer Program
Division Hematology / Oncology
Scottsdale
Phone: 602 301-7504

Mark H. Green, MD
Mayo Clinic
Scottsdale
Contact: Julie Braaten
Phone: 602 301-7050
Fax: 602 301-7155
E-mail: mrb1247@post-ov.mayo.edu

Lois J. Loescher
Arizona Cancer Center
Tucson
Phone: 520 626-7254
Fax: 520 529-3884
E-Mail: loescher@azcc.arizona.edu

Counselors are listed alphabetically by state, city, and name.

Arkansas
*Becky B. Butler, MSSW**
University Arkansas Medical School
Arkansas Genetics Program
Little Rock
Phone: 800 358-7229
Fax: 501 320-1564

Mary A. Curtis, MD
University of Arkansas
for Medical Sciences
Little Rock
Contact: Libby Sexton
Phone: 501 320-2966
Fax: 501 320-1564

California
*Patricia T. Kelly, PhD**
John Muir Medical Center
1601 Ygnacio Valley Road
Walnut Creek
Phone: 510 947-4453
Fax: 510 947-5260

Deborah MacDonald, RN, MS
City of Hope National
Medical Center
Duarte
Phone: 818 359-8111, ext. 4330
Fax: 818 930-5495

*Jeffrey Weitzel, MD**
City of Hope National
Medical Center
Duarte
Phone: 818 359-8111, ext. 4324
Fax: 818 930-5495

Cynthia J. Curry, MD
Valley Children's Hospital-
Medical Genetics
Fresno
Contact: Zohra Ali-Khan
Phone: 209 243-6626
Fax: 209 225-9022
E-Mail: vchgene@cybergate.com

*Tina Bartell, MS**
Loma Linda University
Medical Center
Loma Linda
Phone: 800-78CANCER
Fax: 909 799-6047

*Monica Alvarado, MS**
USC, Norris Comprehensive
Cancer Center
Los Angeles
Phone: 213 764-0800
Fax: 213 764-0102

Robin D. Clark, MD
Norris Comprehensive
Cancer Center
University of Southern California
Los Angeles
Phone: 213 764-0800
Fax: 213 764-0102
E-Mail: clark_r@froggy.hsc.usc.edu

*Karen Klein, PhD**
UCLA Women's
Gyn-Oncology Center
Los Angeles
Phone: 310 794-9096
Fax: 310 794-9110

*Maren T. Scheuner, MD, PhD**
Division of Medical Genetics
Cedars-Sinai Medical Center
Los Angeles
Contact: Helen E. C. Hixon
Phone: 310 855-2211
Fax: 213 651-5381
E-Mail:
hhixon@mailgate.csmc.edu

Ann Bastian
Kaiser Permanente Medical
Center, Oakland
Contact: Genetics Department
Secretary (Kaiser members only)
Phone: 510 596-6298
Fax: 510 596-6754

Ronald Backman, MD
*Kaiser Permanente Medical
Center-Oakland
Contact: Genetics Department
Secretary (Kaiser members only)
Phone: 510 596-6298
Fax: 510 596-6754*

John Baker, MD
*Kaiser Permanente Medical
Center-Oakland
Contact: Genetics Department
Secretary (Kaiser members only)
Phone: 510 596-6298
Fax: 510 596-6754*

*Dawn Banasiak
Kaiser Permanente Medical
Center-Oakland
Contact: Genetics
Department Secretary
(Kaiser members only)
Phone: 510 596-6298
Fax: 510 596-6754*

*Kathy Barnhart
Kaiser Permanente Medical
Center-Oakland
Contact: Genetics Department
Secretary (Kaiser members only)
Phone: 510 596-6298
Fax: 510 596-6754*

Andrea Fishbach, MS, MPH*
*Kaiser Permanente, Colon
Cancer Genetics Program
Oakland
Phone: 510 596-6588
Fax: 510 596-6754*

*Barbara Loebel
Kaiser Permanente Medical
Center-Oakland
Contact: Genetics Department
Secretary (Kaiser members only)
Phone: 510 596-6298
Fax: 510 596-6754*

*Ann Stembridge Kung
Kaiser Permanente Medical
Center Genetics Department-
Oakland
Phone: 510 596-6303
Fax: 510 596-6754
E-mail:
ann.stembridge@ncal.kaiperm.org*

*Barbara Ziel
Kaiser Permanente Medical
Center-Oakland
Contact: Genetics Department
Secretary (Kaiser members only)
Phone: 510 596-6298
Fax: 510 596-6754*

Robert T. Eagan, MD
*St. Joseph Hospital
Regional Cancer Center
Orange
Contact: Debra Treece-Rogriguez or
Jana L. Chavez
Phone: 714 771-8999, ext. 8963
Fax: 714 744-8592*

*Ann P. Walker
Division of Human Genetics
Department of Pediatrics
University of California, Irvine
Orange
Phone: 714 456-5789
Fax: 714 456-5330
E-Mail: awalker@uci.edu*

Faye A. Eggerding, MD, PhD
*Huntington Medical
Research Institutes
Pasadena
Phone: 818 795-4343
Fax: 818 795-5774
E-Mail: eggerdfa@hmri.org*

Ellen Knell, PhD*
*Pasadena
Phone: 818 405-1900
Fax: 818 683-3932*

Linda Marie Randolpf, MD
Alfigen / The Genetics Institute
Pasadena
Contact: Francesca Holland
Phone: 818 666-1337
Fax: 818 795-1948

Shelly Levin, MS*
Kaiser Permanente
Genetics Department
Sacramento
Phone: 916 978-1402
Fax: 916 978-1515

Kimberly Barr
Kaiser Permanente
Genetics Department
San Francisco
Contact: Genetics Department
Secretary (Kaiser members only)
Phone: 415 202-2998
Fax: 415 202-2999

Sandra Blum, BA*
University of California
San Francisco
Phone: 415 885-7481

Bruce Blumberg, MD
Kaiser Permanente Genetics
Department
San Francisco
Contact: Genetics Department
Secretary (Kaiser members only)
Phone: 415 202-2998
Fax: 415 202-2999

Norma Chow
Kaiser Permanente Genetics
Department-San Francisco
Contact: Genetics Department
Secretary (Kaiser members only)
Phone: 415 202-2998
Fax: 415 202-2999

*Beth B. Crawford**
UCSF Mt. Zion Cancer
Risk Program
San Francisco
Phone: 415 885-7779
Fax: 415 885-7218
E-mail:
beth_crawford@quickmail.ucsf.edu

Kathy Culver
Kaiser Permanente Genetics
Department-San Francisco
Contact: Genetics Department
Secretary (Kaiser members only)
Phone: 415 202-2998
Fax: 415 202-2999

Kathleen Fergus
Kaiser Permanente Genetics
Department-San Francisco
Contact: Genetics Department
Secretary (Kaiser members only)
Phone: 415 202-2998
Fax: 415 202-2999

Nancy Hanson
Kaiser Permanente Genetics
Department-San Francisco
Contact: Genetics Department
Secretary (Kaiser members only)
Phone: 415 202-2998
Fax: 415 202-2999

Christine Hartlove
Kaiser Permanente Genetics
Department-San Francisco
Contact: Genetics Department
Secretary (Kaiser members only)
Phone: 415 202-2998
Fax: 415 202-2999

Kathleen Johnston, MD
Kaiser Permanente Genetics
Department-San Francisco
Contact: Genetics Department
Secretary (Kaiser members only)
Phone: 415 202-2998
Fax: 415 202-2999

Kristina Keilman, MS
Kaiser Permanente Genetics
Department-San Francisco
Contact: Genetics Department
Secretary (Kaiser members only)
Phone: 415 202-2998
Fax: 415 202-2999

Amy Vance
Kaiser Permanente Genetics
Department-San Francisco
Contact: Genetics Department
Secretary (Kaiser members only)
Phone: 415 202-2998
Fax: 415 202-2999

*Nicki Chun, MS**
Stanford Medical Center
Stanford
Phone: 415 723-6858
Fax: 415 723-2097

Jerome B. Block, MD
Division of Medical Oncology,
Torrance
Harbor-UCLA Medical Center
Phone: 310 222-2443
Fax: 310 782-0486

*Angela M. Musial, MS**
Alfigen-The Genetics Institute
Walnut Creek
Phone: 510 937-0620
Fax: 510 937-5936

Colorado
*Lisa Mullineaux, MBA, MS**
University of Colorado
Cancer Center
Denver
Phone: 303 372-9113
Fax: 303 372-9129

*Jeffrey Shaw, MS**
Penrose Cancer Center
Herditary Cancer Service
Colorado Springs
Phone: 719 776-5274
Fax: 719 776-2516

Bethany D. Tucker
University of Colorado
Cancer Center
Denver
Contact: Cindy Braden
Phone: 1-800-473-2288 or
303 329-3066
Fax: 303 315-7163

Connecticut
*Robert Pilarski, MS**
Connecticut Children's
Medical Center
Hartford
Phone: 860 545-9578
Fax: 860 545-9590

*Ellen Matloff, MS**
Yale University School
of Medicine
New Haven
Phone: 203 785-5938
Fax: 203 785-7673

*Jennifer L. Scalia, MS**
The Stamford Hospital
Bennett Cancer Center
Stamford
Phone: 203 325-7693
Fax: 203 967-5960

District of Columbia
See Washington, District of Columbia

Florida
*Jennifer Schmidt, MS**
Alfigen Genetics Center
of South Florida
Coral Springs
Phone: 954 255-9771
Fax: 954 255-9772

Edith A. Perez, MD
Mayo Clinic
Jacksonville
Contact: M. Cathie Smith
Phone: 904 953-7290
Fax: 904 953-2315

Carolyn C. Gilleland
Columbia Cedars Medical Center
Miami
Contact: Elizabeth Anne Groh
Phone: 305 325-5769
Fax: 305 325-4549

*Danielle LaGrave, MS**
Orlando Regional Health
Care System
Orlando
Phone: 407 841-5111, x5859

*Daniel Lee Riconda**
M. D. Anderson Cancer
Center-Orlando/Arnold
Palmer Hospital
Phone: 407 649-6910, x1050
Fax: 407 872-7739

*Terry Diamond, MS**
H. Lee Moffitt Cancer
& Research Center
Tampa
Phone: 813 979-6769 x6981
Fax: 813 979-6758

Rebecca Sutphen, MD
H. Lee Moffitt Cancer and
Research Center
Tampa
Contact: Theresa M. Diamond
Phone: 813 979-6769, x6981
Fax: 813 979-6758

Georgia
Paul G. McDonough, MD
Medical College of Georgia
Augusta
Contact: Ellen E. Parker
Phone: 706 721-2828
Fax: 706 721-6830
E-Mail; eparker@mail.mcg.edu

*Ellen Parker, MS**
Medical College of Georgia
Augusta
Phone: 706 721-2828
Fax: 706 721-6830

Hawaii
*Susan Seto Donlon, MS**
Kapiolani Women's Center
Honolulu
Phone: 808 973-6531
Fax: 808 973-6537

Illinois
Susan V. Hailbeck
Joint Practice Associates
Elmhurst
Phone: 630 941-8032
Fax: 630 941-8432

*Dawn C. Allain, MS**
Cook County Hospital
Chicago
Phone: 312 633-7768
Fax: 312 633-7769

Shelly A. Cummings, MS
University of Chicago
Medical Center
Chicago
Phone: 312 702-4749
Fax: 312 702-0963

Aimee Wonderlick, MS*
Northwestern Memorial
Hospital
Chicago
Phone: 312 908-5737
Fax: 312 908-0806

Judith L. Miller, MS*
University of Illinois
College of Medicine
Peoria
Phone: 309 655-4648
Fax: 309 655-2565

Iowa
Joy Larsen Haidle, MS*
University Hospital School
Iowa City
Phone: 319 353-6133
Fax: 319 353-6933

Indiana
Emily C. Brown
Regional Cancer Center
Cancer Genetics Program
Indianapolis
Phone: 317 841-5656
Fax: 317 351-7813

Cindy Hunter, MS*
Indiana University, Medical and
Molecular Genetics Department
Indianapolis
Phone: 317 274-3060
Fax: 317 274-2387

Emily Lichtenberg, MS*
Indiana Regional Cancer Center
The Center for Genetic Counseling
Indianapolis
Phone: 317 841-5708
Fax: 317 588-7863

Gail Habegger Vance, MD
Department of Medical and
Molecular Genetics
Indianapolis
Indiana University School
of Medicine
Contact: Cindy Dale
Phone: 317 274-2241
Fax: 317 274-2387

Kansas
Debra L. Collins, MS*
Genetics Education Center
University of Kansas
Medical Center
Kansas City
Phone: 913 588-6043
Fax: 913 588-4060

Kentucky
Dawn M. Valasky, MS*
University of Kentucky
Lexington
Phone: 606 257-1594
Fax: 606 323-1931

Louisiana
Leslie Colvin, MSc*
Louisiana State University Medical
Center, Children's Hospital
New Orleans
Phone: 504 896-9254
Fax: 504 896-9410

*Kelly Jackson, MS**
Tulane University School of
Medicine, Human
Genetics Program
New Orleans
Phone: 504 588-5229
Fax: 504 584-1763

Maryland
*Barbara A. Bernhardt, MS**
Johns Hopkins University
Baltimore
Phone: 410 955-7894
Fax: 410 955-0241

*Jill D. Brensinger, MS**
Johns Hopkins University
Baltimore
Phone: 410 614-4038
Fax: 410 614-4038

Karen A. Johnson
Johns Hopkins University
Baltimore
Phone: 410 614-0378
Fax: 410 955-0863
E-mail:
kjohnson@phnet.spu.jhu.edu

*Cari Long, MS**
Greater Baltimore
Medical Center
Baltimore
Phone: 410 828-3131
Fax: 410 828-2919

Gloria M. Petersen, PhD
Johns Hopkins University School
of Public Health
Baltimore
Contact: Karen A. Johnson
Phone: 410 614-0378
Fax: 410 955-0863

Sandra Yang
University of Maryland
Baltimore
Phone: 410 328-3338
Fax: 410 328-3379

*Barbara Bowles Biesecker, MS**
National Human Genome
Research Institute
Bethesda
National Institutes of Health
Phone: 301 496-3979
Fax: 301 496-7157
E-Mail: barbarab@nchgr.nih.gov

Eileen P. Dimond
National Human Genome
Research Institute
Bethesda
National Institutes of Health
Phone: 301 496-0921
Fax: 301 496-0047
E-mail:
dimonde@navmed.nci.nih.gov

Donald W. Hadley
National Human
Genome Research Institute
Bethesda
National Institutes of Health
Contact: Eileen P. Dimond
Phone: 301 496-0921
Fax: 301 496-0047

*June Peters, MS**
National Human Genome
Research Institute
Bethesda
National Institutes of Health
Phone: 301 594-2951
Fax: 301 402-2672

*Joan Scott, MS**
OncorMed, Inc.
Gaithersburg
Phone: 800 662-6763 x546
Fax: 301 926-6125

*Paula Glauber, MS, RN, OCN**
OncorMed, Inc.
Gaithersburg
Phone: 800 662-6763 x546
Fax: 301 926-6125

*Ann Garrity Carr, MS**
Center for Medical Genetics
Rockville
Phone: 301 460-GENE
Fax: 301 517-4999

Massachusetts
*Anu Chittenden, MS**
Dana Farber Cancer Institute
Family Studies Coordinator
Boston
Phone: 617 632-4757
Fax: 617 632-3161

*Elaine Hiller, MS**
Dana Farber Cancer Institute
Boston
Phone: 617 632-2178
Fax: 617 632-3161

*Stephanie A. Kieffer, MS**
Dana Farber Cancer Institute
Boston
Phone: 617 632-2271
Fax: 617 632-3161

*Kristen Mahoney, MS**
Massachusetts General Hospital
Boston
Phone: 617 726-7803
Fax: 617 726-9210

*Susan Mecsas-Faxon, MS**
Harvard Pilgrim Health Plan
Boston
Phone: 617 859-5151
Fax: 617 267-8203

Fredrica A. Preston
North Shore Cancer Center
Peabody
Phone: 508 977-3434
Fax: 508 977-4985

Constance A. Roche
Lahey Hitchcock Clinic
Peabody
Phone: 508 538-4670
Fax: 508 538-4708

*Lori Ann Correia, MS**
Baystate Medical Center
Springfield
Phone: 413 784-8890
Fax: 413 784-8166

Michigan
Thomas D. Gelehrter, MD
Division of Molecular Medicine
and Genetics
University of Michigan
Ann Arbor
Contact: Wendy R. Ulhmann
Phone: 313 763-2532
Fax: 313 763-7672
E-Mail: wuhlmann@umich.edu

David Ginsburg, MD
Division of Molecular Medicine
and Genetics
University of Michigan
Ann Arbor
Contact: Wendy R. Ulhmann
Phone: 313 763-2532
Fax: 313 763-7672
E-Mail: wuhlmann@umich.edu

Virginia M. LeClaire
Comprehensive Cancer Center
University of Michigan
Ann Arbor
Phone: 313 763-3034
Fax: 313 763-6236
E-Mail: vmartin@umich.edu

Jane M. Nicholson, MD
Division of Molecular Medicine
and Genetics
University of Michigan
Ann Arbor
Contact: Wendy R. Ulhmann
Phone: 313 763-2532
Fax: 313 763-7672
E-Mail: wuhlmann@umich.edu

Elizabeth M. Petty, MD
Division of Molecular Medicine
and Genetics
University of Michigan
Ann Arbor
Contact: Wendy R. Ulhmann
Phone: 313 763-2532
Fax: 313 763-7672
E-Mail: wuhlmann@umich.edu

Kelly Taylor, MS*
University of Michigan
Comprehensive Cancer Center
Breast and Ovarian Cancer Risk
Evaluation Program
Ann Arbor
Phone: 313 764-2248
Fax: 313 763-4151

Wendy Uhlmann, MS
University of Michigan
Ann Arbor
Phone: 313 763-2532
Fax: 313 763-7672
E-Mail: wuhlmann@umich.edu

Kate Sargent, MS
Karmanos Cancer Institute
Wertz Outreach
Detroit
Phone: 313 966-7780

Minnesota
Diane Bierke-Nelson, MS, MSSW
Duluth Clinic
Duluth
Phone: 218 725-3012
Fax: 218 722-0170

Thomas T. Amatruda, MD
Familial Cancer Clinic
University of Minnesota
Minneapolis
Contact: Mary J. Ahrens
Phone: 612 625-2134
Fax: 612 624-6645

Mary Ahrens, MS*
University of Minnesota
Minneapolis
Phone: 612 625-2134
Fax: 612 624-6645

Shari Baldinger, MS*
Abbott Northwestern Hospital
Minneapolis
Phone: 612 863-4502
Fax: 612 863-5697

Richard A. King, MD, PhD
Familial Cancer Clinic
University of Minnesota
Minneapolis
Contact: Mary J. Ahrens
Phone: 612 625-2134
Fax: 612 624-6645

Anna Leninger, MS*
Minnesota Department of Health,
Cancer Control Section
Minneapolis
Phone: 612 623-5761
Fax: 612 623-5520

Richard M. Goldberg, MD
Mayo Clinic
Rochester
Contact: Michelle Weber
Phone: 507 286-0029
Fax: 507 284-1803
E-Mail: weber.michelle@mayo.edu

Cate Walsh-Vockley, MS*
Mayo Clinic
Rochester
Department of Medical Genetics
Phone: 507 284-8198
Fax: 507 284-1067

Trine Shimoto, MS
United Hospital
St. Paul
Phone: 612 220-6270
Fax: 612 220-5185

Missouri

Sukmar Ethirajan, MD
Cancer Prevention Clinic
Trinity Lutheran Hospital
Kansas City
Contact: Amy Strauss Tranin
Phone: 816 751-2800
Fax: 816 751-4391
E-Mail: amytranin@wow.com

Amy Strauss Tranin, BSN, MS*
Cancer Prevention Clinic
Trinity Lutheran Hospital
Kansas City
Phone: 816 751-2800
Fax: 816 751-4391
E-Mail: amytranin@wow.com

Sheri A. Babb, MS*
Washington University
School of Medicine
St. Louis
Phone: 314 362-3300
Fax: 314 362-8644

H. Marvin Camel, MD
Washington University
School of Medicine
St. Louis
Contact: Sheri A. Babb
Phone: 314 362-3300
Fax: 314 362-8644

David Ciske
Division of Medical Genetics
Washington University
School of Medicine
St. Louis
Contact: Jennifer Ivanovich
Phone: 314 454-6093
Fax: 314 454-2075

Ruth A. Decker, MD
The Decker Foundation
St. Louis
Phone: 1 800 432-8087
Fax: 314 469-0744

Al Elbendary, MD
Washington University
School of Medicine
St. Louis
Contact: Sheri A. Babb
Phone: 314 362-3300
Fax: 314 362-8644

Thomas Herzog, MD
Washington University
School of Medicine
St. Louis
Contact: Sheri A. Babb
Phone: 314 362-3300
Fax: 314 362-8644

Jennifer Ivanovich, MS*
Division of Medical Genetics
Washington University
School of Medicine
St. Louis
Phone: 314 454-6093
Fax: 314 454-2075

David G Mutch, MD
Washington University
School of Medicine
St. Louis
Contact: Sheri A. Babb
Phone: 314 362-3300
Fax: 314 362-8644

Linda Piersall
Washington University
School of Medicine
St. Louis
Contact: Jennifer Ivanovich
Phone: 314 454-6093
Fax: 314 454-2075

Janet S. Rader, MD
Washington University
School of Medicine
St. Louis
Contact: Sheri A. Babb
Phone: 314 362-3300
Fax: 314 362-8644

Rachel Slaugh
Washington University
School of Medicine
St. Louis
Contact: Jennifer Ivanovich
Phone: 314 454-6093
Fax: 314 454-2075

Alison Whelan, MD
Washington University
School of Medicine
St. Louis
Contact: Jennifer Ivanovich
Phone: 314 454-6093
Fax: 314 454-2075

Montana
John P. Johnson, MD
Medical Genetics
Shodair Hospital
Helena
Contact: Shelly Hammer
Phone: 406 444-7587
Fax: 406 444-7536
E-Mail: shammer@initco.net

Nebraska
Carolyn S. Durham
Hereditary Cancer Institute
Creighton University
Omaha
Phone: 402 280-2634
Fax: 402 280-1734
E-mail: cdurham@creighton.edu

Barbara A. Franklin
Department of Preventive
Medicine
Creighton University
Omaha
Phone: 402 280-2919
Fax: 402 280-1734
E-mail: bfrank@creighton.edu

Marsha B. Karr
Department of
Preventive Medicine
Creighton University
Omaha
Phone: 402 280-2688
Fax: 402 280-1734
E-mail: bkarr@creighton.edu

Stephen J. Lemon, MD
Department of
Preventive Medicine
Creighton University
Omaha
Contact: Susan T. Tinley
Phone: 402 280-1796
Fax: 402 280-1734
E-mail: tinley@creighton.edu

*Henry T. Lynch, MD**
Creighton University
School of Medicine
Omaha
Phone: 402 280-2942
Fax: 402 280-1734

Gwendolyn M. Reiser
Hereditary Cancer Clinic
U. Nebraska Medical Center
Omaha
Phone: 402 559-4161
Fax: 402 559-7248
E-mail: greiser@unmc.edu

Carrie L. Snyder
Department of
Preventive Medicine
Creighton University
Omaha
Phone: 402 280-2634
Fax: 402 280-1734
E-mail: csnyder@creighton.edu

Susan T. Tinley
Hereditary Cancer Prevention
Clinic
Creighton University
Omaha
Phone: 402 280-1796
Fax: 402 280-1734

New Hampshire
Bradley A. Arrick, MD, PhD
Norris Cotton Cancer Center
Dartmouth Medical School
Hanover
Phone: 603 650-1550
Fax: 603 650-7791
E-mail:
bradley.arrick@dartmouth.edu

New Jersey
Patty M. Barse
Cooper Hospital / University
Medical Center
Camden
Phone: 609 963-3572
Fax: 609 338-9211

*Sivya Twersky, MS**
Hackensack University
Medical Center
Hackensack
Phone: 201 996-5264
Fax: 201 996-0827

*Judy Rokeach, RN**
Monmouth Medical Center
Jacqueline Wilenz Comprehensive
Breast Center
Long Beach
Phone: 909 222-5200 x5360

*Michelle B. Horner, MS**
St. Peter's Medical Center
New Brunswick
Phone: 908 745-6659
Fax: 908 249-2687

Nita Patel
Institute of Clinical Genetics
St. Peter's Medical Center
New Brunswick
Phone: 908 745-6659
Fax: 908 249-2687

*Monica Magee, MS**
UMDNJ, Center for Human and
Molecular Genetics
Newark
Phone: 201 982-3300
Fax: 201 982-3310

Suzanne M. DiStaso
Community Medical Center
Toms River
Phone: 908 240-8107
Fax: 908 240-8952

New York
Karen Greendale, MA*
New York State Department
of Health, Wadsworth Center
Albany
Phone: 518 473-8036
Fax: 518 473-1733
Resource referrals only. Does not
see patients or conduct research.

Kathy Keenan, MS*
The Women's Health Center
of Albany Medical Center
Hereditary Breast and Ovarian
Cancer Screening Program
Albany
Phone: 518 464-0084
Fax: 518 262-5292

John H. Malfetano, MD
Department of Obstetrics/
Gynecology
Albany Medical College
Albany
Contact: Ann B. Murphy
Phone: 518 262-5260
Fax: 518 262-4964

Luba Djurdjinovic, MS*
Genetic Counseling Program
Binghamton
Phone: 607 724-4308
Fax: 607 724-8290

Myrna Ben-Yishay*
Reproductive Genetics
Bronx
Phone: 718 405-8150
Fax: 718 405-8154
E-mail: mby14@aol.com

Robert D. Burk, MD
Albert Einstein College
of Medicine
Bronx
Phone: 718 430-3720
Fax: 718 430-8975
E-mail: burk@aecom.yu.edu

Howard J. Allen, PhD, MSW*
Roswell Park Cancer Institute
Buffalo
Phone: 716 845-5725
Fax: 716 845-3458

Carolyn Farrell, MS, CNP*
Roswell Park Cancer Institute
Buffalo
Phone: 716 845-7747
Fax: 716 845-3434

Mary-Jo Tout Rosenblatt, MS*
Roswell Park Cancer Institute
Clinical Genetics Service
Buffalo
Phone: 716 845-8400
Fax: 716 845-3434

Tammy P. Snell, MS*
Cancer Center at Glens
Falls Hospital
Glens Falls
Phone: 518 742-2920
Fax: 518 761-2208

Carrie McKenna
Child Development
& Human Genetics
North Shore
University Hospital
Manhasset
Phone: 516 365-3996
Fax: 516 365-4597

*Lauren Scheuer, MS**
North Shore University Hospital
Manhasset
Phone: 516 926-4357

*Karen L. Brown, MS**
Memorial Sloan-Kettering
Cancer Center
Clinical Genetics Service
New York
Phone: 212 639-6760
Fax: 212 717-3129

*Mary Kay Dabney, MS**
Strang Cancer Prevention Center
New York
Phone: 212 794-4900 x111
Fax: 212 794-4958

Randolph E. Gross
Special Surveillance Breast
Program
Memorial Sloan-Kettering
Cancer Center
New York
Phone: 212 639-5250
Fax: 212 319-2284

*Bruce R. Haas, MS**
Memorial Sloan-Kettering Cancer
Center
Clinical Genetics Service
New York
Phone: 212 639-6760
Fax: 212 717-3129

*Heather Hampel, MS**
Memorial Sloan-Kettering Cancer
Center, Clinical Genetics Service
New York
Phone: 212 639-6760
Fax: 212 717-3129

Kenneth Offit, MD
Contact: Cicely Corbett
Memorial Sloan-Kettering
Cancer Center
New York
Phone: 212 639-6760
Fax: 212 717-3129

*Elisa Reich, MS**
New York University
School of Medicine
Human Genetics Program
New York
Phone: 212 263-6603
Fax: 212 263-7590

*Gladys Rosenthal, MS**
Strang Cancer
Prevention Center
New York
Phone: 212 794-4900 x120
Fax: 212 794-4958

*Donna Russo, MS**
Columbia-Presbyterian
Medical Center
New York
Phone: 212 305-0190
Fax: 212 305-1522

*Charlene Schulz, MS**
Memorial Sloan-Kettering
Cancer Center
New York
Phone: 212 639-6760
Fax: 212 717-3129

Melanie K. McDermet
L.I. Regional Genetics Program
Central Suffolk Hospital
Riverhead
Phone: 516 548-6866
Fax: 516 548-6853

Peter T. Rowley, MD
Division of Genetics
U. Rochester School of Medicine
Rochester
Contact: Starlene Loader
Phone: 716 275-4602
Fax: 716 273-1034
E-mail:
sloader@medicine.rochester.edu

Beth Siegel, MS*
The Genetics Center
Smithtown
Phone: 516 862-3620
Fax: 516 862-3622

North Carolina
Kerry Crandell, MS*
Mission Genetic Center
Asheville
Phone: 704 252-7037
Fax: 704 252-6954

Philip D. Buchanan, PhD
GeneCare Medical
Genetics Center
Chapel Hill
Contact: Ruth G. Scherer
Phone: 800 277-4363
Fax: 919 967-9519
E-mail: genecare@earthlink.net

Cecile Skrzynia, MS*
University of North
Carolina-Chapel Hill
Phone: 919 966-4431
Fax: 919 966-6735

Lisa Amacker North, MS*
Carolinas Medical Center
Charlotte
Phone: 704 355-3159
Fax: 704 355-8700

Julie Jackson Sawyer, MS*
Presbyterian Hospital
Charlotte
Phone: 704 384-5908
Fax: 704 384-5642

W. Abe Andes, MD
Comprehensive Cancer Center
of Wake Forest University
Winston-Salem
Phone: 910 716-4922
Fax: 910 716-3671

Daragh Marnane, MS*
Bowman Gray School of Medicine
Winston-Salem
Phone: 901 716-2213
Fax: 901 716-7100

Ohio
Karen Huelsman, MS*
Children's Hospital Medical Center
The Hereditary Cancer Program
Cincinnati
Phone: 513 636-4760
Fax: 513 636-7297

Howard M. Saal, MD
Hereditary Cancer Program
Division of Human Genetics
Cincinnati
Contact: Karen M. Huelsman
Phone: 513 559-5576, x3871
Fax: 513 559-7297
E-mail: huelk0@chmcc.org

Brian A. Clark, MD, PhD
Cleveland Clinic Foundation
Cleveland
Contact: Linda S. Webster
Phone: 216 445-5686
Fax: 216 445-6935
E-mail: webstel@mintaka.cc.ccf.org

Rebecca J. Shrigley
Center for Human Genetics
University Hospitals of Cleveland
Cleveland
Phone: 216 844-3936
Fax: 216 844-7497
E-mail: rjs15@po.cwru.edu

Georgia L. Wiesner, MD
Center for Human Genetics
University Hospitals
of Cleveland
Cleveland
Phone: 216-844-3936
Fax: 216-844-7497
E-mail: rjs15@po.cwru.edu

Judith A. Westman, MD
Arthur G. James Cancer Hospital
& Research Institute
Columbus
Contact: Jennifer S. Graham
Phone: 614 293-6694
Fax: 614 293-2314
E-mail: graham-
1@medctr.osu.edu

Faith A. Callif-Daley
Children's Medical Center
Dayton
Phone: 937 226-8408
Fax: 937 463-5325
E-mail: fcdgc@aol.com

Marvin E. Miller, MD
Children's Medical Center
Dayton
Contact: Faith A. Callif-Daley
Phone: 937 226-8408
Fax: 937 463-5325
E-mail: fcdgc@aol.com

Oklahoma
Alan B. Hollingsworth, MD
Institute for Breast Health
U. Oklahoma Health
Sciences Center
Oklahoma City
Contact: Barbara J. Holmberg
Phone: 405 271-4514
Fax: 405271-3495

Frederick V. Schaefer, PhD
H.A. Chapman Institute
of Medical Genetics
Tulsa
Phone: 918 628-6363
Fax: 918 664-0596

Oregon
Kathryn Murray, MS*
Sacred Heart General
Eugene
Phone: 541 686-7419
Fax: 541 686-8330

Lisa C. Wisniewski
Emanuel Hospital
and Health Center
Portland
Phone: 800 452-7032, x34726
Fax: 503 413-2829

Pennsylvania
Thomas G. Frazier, MD
The Diagnostic Breast Center
Bryn Mawr
Phone: 610 520-0700
Fax: 610 520-0744

Josephine Costalas, MS*
Fox Chase Cancer Center
Cheltenham
Phone: 215 728-2727
Fax: 215 728-4061

Mary B. Daly, MD, PhD
Fox Chase Cancer Center
Cheltenham
Contact: Joanne Spoltore
Phone: 800 325-4145
Fax: 215 728-2707
E-mail: j_spotore@fccc.edu

Susan V. Montgomery
Fox Chase Cancer Center
Cheltenham
Contact: Mary B. Daly, MD, PhD
Phone: 215 728-2705
Fax: 215 728-2707

Elizabeth A. Kopp
Pinnacle Health Regional
Cancer Center
Harrisburg
Phone: 717 782-2655
Fax: 717 782-2957

Kathleen A. Calzone
U. Pennsylvania Cancer Center
Philadelphia
Phone: 215 349-8141
Fax: 215 662-7617
E-mail:
calzone@mail.med.upenn.edu

*Lynn Godmilow, MSW**
University of Pennsylvania
School of Medicine
Philadelphia
Phone: 215 573-9161
Fax: 215 573-7760

Donna C. Goodwin
Division of Medical Genetics
Thomas Jefferson University
Philadelphia
Contact: Laird G. Jackson, MD
Phone: 215 955-5080
Fax: 215 955-7560

Lisa K. Jablon, MD
Albert Einstein Medical Center
Philadelphia
Phone: 215 456-8722
Fax: 215 456-2356
E-mail: aemcgenetics@icdc.com

Lisa S. Steinberg
Albert Einstein Medical Center
Philadelphia
Phone: 215 456-8722
Fax: 215 456-2356
E-mail: aemcgenetics@icdc.com

*Jill Stopfer, MS**
University Hospital of Pennsylvania
Breast / Ovarian Cancer Risk
Evaluation Program
Phone: 215 898-0247
Colon Cancer Risk
Evaluation Program
Philadelphia
Phone: 215 662-4740
Fax: 215 662-7617

*Betsy Gettig, MS**
University of Pennsylvania
Department of Genetics
Pittsburgh
Phone: 412 624-9951
Fax: 412 624-3020

*Sandra Marchese, MS**
Alleghany General Hospital,
Center for Human Genetics
Pittsburgh
Phone: 412 359-4485
Fax: 412 359-6488

John J. Mulvihill, MD
Cancer Genetics Program
University of Pittsburgh
Pittsburgh
Contact: Mona P. Stadler
Phone: 800-454-8156
Fax: 412 621-1032

*Wendy S. Rubinstein, MD, PhD**
Comprehensive Breast
Cancer Program
U. Pittsburgh Cancer Institute
Pittsburgh
Phone: 412 692-2620
Fax: 412 692-2610

*Mona P. Stadler, MS**
Magee Women's Hospital
Cancer Genetics Program
Pittsburgh
Phone: 800 454-8156
Fax: 412 641-1032

*Darcy Thull, MS**
Alleghany General Hospital
Center for Human Genetics
Pittsburgh
Phone: 412 359-4485
Fax: 412 359-6488

*Mary Elaine Southard, RN, MSN**
Northeast Regional Cancer
Institute, University
of Scranton Campus
Scranton
Phone: 717 941-7984
Fax: 717 941-7979

*Laura Toole, MSS, MSLP**
Northeast Regional
Cancer Institute
Scranton
Phone: 717 941-7984
Fax: 717 941-7979

Stanley J. Yamulla, MD
Phone: 717 455-5864
Fax: 717 455-0546

South Carolina
G. Shashidhar Pai, MD
Division of Genetics
Medical University
of South Carolina
Charleston
Contact: Loy Ballam
Phone: 800 424-6872 or
803 792-7137
Fax: 803 792-3597
E-mail: ballaml@musc.edu

*Karen Brooks, MS**
University of South Carolina
School of Medicine
Columbia
Phone: 803 779-4928 x229
Fax: 803 434-7756

*Angela Tutera, MS**
University of South
Carolina School of Medicine
Columbia
Phone: 803 779-4928 x270
Fax: 803 434-7756

*S. Robert Young, PhD**
University of South Carolina
Columbia
Phone: 803 779-4928
Fax: 803 434-4699
E-mail: young-sr@sc.edu

*Judith Lax Green, MSW**
Mt. Pleasant
Phone: 803 881-8346

Tennessee
*Maureen E. Smith**
Baptist Cancer Institute
Memphis
Phone: 901 227-7465
Fax: 901 227-0035
E-mail: maureenes@aol.com

Susan W. Caro
Vanderbilt University
Medical Center
Nashville
Phone: 615 322-2064
Fax: 615 343-0746
E-mail:
carosw@ctrvax.vanderbilt.edu

*Melinda Cohen, MS**
Vanderbilt University
Medical Center
Nashville
Phone: 615 322-7601
Fax: 615 343-9951

Texas
*Karen Copeland, MS**
Central Texas Genetics Center
Austin
Phone: 512 451-5173
Fax: 512 459-0846

Gail S. Brookshire
Children's Medical Center
Dallas
Contact: Kristin Shelby
Phone: 214 648-8539
Fax: 214 648-2792

*Karen Heller, MS**
Genetic Counseling Associates
Dallas
Phone: 972 458-8699
Fax: 972 458-9060

Gail E. Tomlinson, MD, PhD
U.T. Southwestern Medical Center
Dallas
Contact: Kristin Shelby
Phone: 214 648-8539
Fax: 214 648-2792

Laura L. Rice
M.D. Anderson Cancer Network
Tarrant County
Fort Worth
Phone: 817 820-4864
Fax: 817 820-4890

Robert F. Gagel, MD
U.T. M.D. Anderson Cancer Center
Houston
Contact: Pamela N. Schultz
Phone: 713-792-2840
Fax: 713-794-4065
E-mail:
pam_schultz@isqm.mda.uth.tmc.edu

Patrick M. Lynch, JD, MD
U.T. M.D. Anderson Cancer Center
Houston
Contact: Jill C. Sawyer
Phone: 713 745-2385
Fax: 713 794-4730
E-mail:
jsawyer@notes.mdacc.tmc.edu

Gordon B. Mills, MD, PhD
U.T. M.D. Anderson Cancer Center
Houston
Contact: Paula T. Rieger
Phone: 713 745-8040
Fax: 713 745-8046
E-mail:
prieger@notes.mdacc.tmc.edu

Paula T. Rieger
U.T. M.D. Anderson Cancer Center
Houston
Phone: 713 745-8040
Fax: 713 745-8046

*Jill Sawyer, MS**
U.T. M.D. Anderson Cancer Center
Houston
Phone: 713 745-2385
Fax: 713 794-4730

Sheila Dobin, PhD
Scott and White Clinic
Temple
Contact: Rebecca L. Finkbohner
Phone: 817 742-3700
Fax: 817 742-3705
E-mail: smdobin@tamu.edu

Utah
*Susan Manley, MS**
Myriad Genetics
Salt Lake City
Phone: 801 584-3505
Fax: 801 584-3515

*Jamie McDonald, MS**
Huntsman Cancer Institute
University of Utah Medical Center
Salt Lake City
Phone: 801 585-2579
Fax: 801 585-5763

*Vickie L. Venne, MS**
Huntsman Cancer Institute
Salt Lake City
Phone: 801 585-7364
Fax: 801 585-6763
E-mail:
marybeth.hart@genetics.utah.edu

Vermont
*Wendy C. McKinnon**
Familial Cancer Program of the
Vermont Cancer Center
Burlington
Phone: 802 658-4310
Fax: 802 860-7542
E-mail:
mckinnon@salus.med.uvm.edu

Virginia
*Susan M. Jones, MS**
UVA Health Science Cancer Center
Charlottesville
Phone: 804 243-6446
Fax: 804 982-0918

Joann N. Bodurtha, MD
Medical College of Virginia
Richmond
Contact: Steve Rice
Phone: 804 828-9632
Fax: 804 828-3760
E-mail: service@gems.vcu.edu

David Trent, MD, PhD
Columbia Henrico
Doctors Hospital
Richmond
Contact: Abbi J. Bruce
Phone: 804 285-5174
Fax: 804 285-5189

Washington
*Julie O. Bars, MS**
University of Washington
Seattle
Phone: 206 616-4978
Fax: 206 616-4302

*Robin L. Bennett, MS**
University of Washington
Medical Center, Medical Genetics
Seattle
Phone: 206 548-4030
Fax: 206 616-4196

*Jamie Dann, MS**
University of Washington
Mary Claire King Laboratory
Seattle
Phone: 206 616-4293
Fax: 206 616-4295

Erin D. Ellis, MD
The Swedish Breast Cancer Center
Contact: Sandra J. Coe
Seattle
Phone: 206 386-2101
Fax: 206 386-2555

Susie Ball
Genetics - Memorial Hospital
Yakima
Phone: 509 575-8160
Fax: 509 577-5088
E-mail: susieball@aol.com

Washington,
District of Columbia
Michelle E. Martin, MS*
Columbia Hospital for Women
Division of Reproductive Genetics
Washington, DC
Phone: 202 293-4944
Fax: 202 778-6203

Beth N. Peshkin, MS*
Georgetown University
Medical Center
Washington, DC
Phone: 202 687-1750
Fax: 202 687-0820

Jeri E. Reutenauer
Lombardi Cancer Center
Georgetown U. Medical Center
Washington, DC
Contact: Jennifer Rocca
Phone: 202 687-1750
Fax: 202 687-0820
E-mail:
roccaj@gunet.georgetown.edu

Wisconsin
Sumedha Ghate, MS*
St. Vincent Hospital, Perinatal
Services-Genetics
Green Bay
Phone: 414 433-8634 or
800 236-3030 x8634
Fax: 414 431-3126

Peter J. Levonian, MS*
Gundersen Lutheran
Familial Cancer Program
LaCrosse
Phone: 608 782-7300 x3995
Fax: 608 791-6361

Kristin M. Baker
Meriter Hospital
Madison
Contact: Margo Grady
Phone: 608 267-6261
Fax: 608 257-1255
E-mail:
mgrady@meriter.medsch.wisc.edu

Joanne M. Becker, MS*
Wisconsin Clinical
Genetics Center
U. Wisconsin Cancer Center
Madison
Contact: Vickie R. Draeger
Phone: 608 263-2510
Fax: 608 263-3496
E-mail: draeger@waisman.wisc.edu

Cecelia Bellcross, MS*
St. Mary's Medical Center, Dean
Medical Center, Perinatology Clinic
Madison
Phone: 608 258-5697
Fax: 608 258-6772

Margo Grady, MS*
Meriter Hospital
Prenatal Diagnosis Clinic
Madison
Phone: 608 267-6261
Fax: 608 267-6364

V. Kim Horton
Wisconsin Clinical
Genetics Center
U. Wisconsin Comprehensive
Cancer Center
Madison
Contact: Vickie R. Draeger
Phone: 608 263-2510
Fax: 608 263-3496
E-mail:
draeger@waisman.wisc.edu

*Wendy Robertson, MS**
St. Mary's Hospital Medical
Center, Dean Medical Center
Perinatology Clinic
Madison
Phone: 608 252-7458
Fax: 608 258-6772

*Connie Rae Schultz, MS**
St. Mary's Hospital Medical
Center Dean Medical Center,
Perinatology Clinic
Madison
Phone: 608 258-5699
Fax: 608 258-6772

*Kristin Sanden, MS**
Children's Hospital Wisconsin
Milwaukee
Phone: 414 266-3345
Fax: 414 266 2653

CANADA
Alberta
Renee H. Martin, PhD
Alberta Children's Hospital
Calgary
Contact: Michelle Phillips
Phone: 403 229-7373
Fax: 403 229-7371
E-mail: michp@ach.ucalgary.ca

British Columbia
Karen L. Panabaker
British Columbia Cancer Agency
Vancouver
Contact: Mary K. McCullum
Phone: 604 877-6000, x2133
Fax: 604 872-4596
E-mail: mmccullum@bccancer.bc.ca

Patrick M. MacLeod, MD
Victoria General Hospital
Victoria
Phone: 604 727-4461
Fax: 604 727-4295
E-mail: pmacleod@gvhs.gov.bc.ca

Ontario
Helene M.F. Perras
Loeb Medical Research Institute
Ottawa Civic Hospital
Ottawa
Phone: 613 798-5555, x7805
Fax: 613 761-5365
E-mail:
genetics@civich.ottawa.on.ca

Quebec
Lidia Z. Kasprzak
Royal Victoria Hospital
Montreal
Phone: 514 843-1449 or
514 842-1231, x5571
Fax: 514 843-1712
E-mail:
lkasprza@rvhmed.lan.mcgill.ca

*Elizabeth Hoodfar, MS**
Centre for Research
in Women's Health
Toronto
Phone: 416 351-3768
Fax: 416 351-3767

APPENDIX 2

Other Resources for Further Information

American Cancer Society (ACS)
(800) ACS-2345 (8:30 AM–4:30 PM)
1599 Clifton Road, NE
Atlanta, Georgia

ACS—Alabama (Mid-South Division, Inc.): 504 Brookwood Boulevard, Birmingham, AL 35209-6802; 205-879-2242

ACS—Alaska (Western Pacific Division, Inc.): 1057 Fireweed Lane, Suite 204, Anchorage, AK 99503; 907-277-8696

ACS—Arizona (Southwest Division, Inc.): 2929 East Thomas Road, Phoenix, AZ 85016; 602-224-0524

ACS—Arkansas (Mid-South Division, Inc.): 901 North University, Little Rock, AR 72207; 501-664-3480

ACS—California (California Division, Inc.): 1710 Webster Street, Oakland, CA 94612; 510-893-7900

ACS—Colorado (Colorado Division, Inc.): 2255 South Oncida, Denver, CO 80224; 303-758-2030

ACS—Connecticut (Connecticut Division, Inc.): 14 Village Lane—Barnes Park South, Wallingford, CT 06492; 203-265-7161

ACS—Delaware (Mid-Atlantic Division, Inc.): 92 Read's Way, Suite 205, New Castle, DE 19720; 302-324-4227

ACS—District of Columbia (Mid-Atlantic Division, Inc.): 1875 Connecticut Avenue NW, Suite 730, Washington, DC 20009; 202-483-2600

ACS—Florida (Florida Division, Inc.): 3709 West Jetton Avenue, Tampa, FL 33629-5146; 813-253-0541

ACS—Georgia (Georgia Division, Inc.): 2200 Lake Boulevard, Atlanta, GA 30319; 404-816-7800

ACS—Hawaii (Hawaii Pacific Division, Inc.): 2370 Nuuanu Avenue, Honolulu, HI 96817; 808-595-7500

ACS—Idaho (Idaho Division, Inc.): 2676 Vista Avenue, Boise, ID 83705; 208-343-4609

ACS—Illinois (Illinois Division, Inc.): 77 East Monroe Street, Chicago, IL 60603-5795; 312-641-6150

ACS—Indiana (Indiana Division Inc.): 8730 Commerce Park Place, Indianapolis, IN 46268; 317-872-4432

ACS—Iowa (Iowa Division, Inc.): 8364 Hickman Road, Suite D, Des Moines, IA 50325-4300; 515-253-0147

ACS—Kentucky (Mid-South Division, Inc.): 701 West Muhammad Ali Boulevard, Louisville, KY 40203-1909; 502-584-6782

ACS—Las Vegas (Southwest Division, Inc.): 1325 East Harmon, Las Vegas, NV 89119; 702-798-6857

ACS—Louisiana (Mid-South Division, Inc.): 2200 Veterans Memorial Blvd, Suite 214, Kenner, LA 70062; 504-469-0021

ACS—Maine (Maine Division, Inc.): 52 Federal Street, Brunswick, ME 04011; 207-729-3339

ACS—Maryland (Mid-Atlantic Division, Inc.): 8219 Town Center Drive, Baltimore, MD 21236-0026; 410-931-6850

ACS—Massachusetts (Massachusetts Division, Inc.): 30 Speen Street, Framingham, MA 01701-1800; 508-270-4600

ACS—Michigan (Michigan Division, Inc.): 1205 East Saginaw Street, Lansing, MI 48906; 517-371-2920

ACS—Minnesota (Minnesota Division, Inc.): 3316 West 66th Street, Minneapolis, MN 55435; 612-925-2772

ACS—Mississippi (Mid-South Division, Inc.): 1380 Livingston Lane, Jackson, MS 39213; 601-362-8874

ACS—Missouri (Heartland Division, Inc.): 1100 Pennsylvania Avenue, Kansas City, MO 64105; 816-842-7111

ACS—Montana (Montana Division, Inc.): 1 South Montana Avenue, Helena, MT 59601; 406-449-9300

ACS—New Jersey (New Jersey Division, Inc.): 2600 US Highway 1, North Brunswick, NJ 08902-6001; 908-297-8000

ACS—New Hampshire (New Hampshire Division, Inc.): 360 State Route 101, Suite 501, Bedford, NH 03110-5032; 603-472-8899

ACS—New Mexico (Southwest Division, Inc.): 5800 Lomas Boulevard NE, Albuquerque, NM 87110; 505-260-2105

ACS—New York: (5 locations)

(New York State Division, Inc.) 6725 Lyons Street, East Syracuse, NY 13057; 315-437-7025

(Long Island Division, Inc.) 75 Davids Drive, Hauppauge, NY 11788; 516-436-7070

(New York City Division, Inc.) 19 West 56th Street, New York, NY 10019; 212-586-8700

(Westchester Divison, Inc.) 2 Lyon Place, White Plains, NY 10601; 914-949-4800

(Queens Division, Inc.): 112-25 Queens Blvd., Forest Hills, NY 11375; 718-263-2224

ACS—North Carolina (North Carolina Division, Inc.): 11 S. Boylan Avenue, Ste. 221, Raleigh, NC 27603; 919-834-8463

ACS—North Dakota (North Dakota Division, Inc.): 1005 Westrac Drive, Fargo, ND 58103; 701-232-1385

ACS—Ohio (Ohio Division, Inc.): 5555 Franz Road, Dublin, OH 43017; 614-889-9565

ACS—Oregon (Oregon Division, Inc.): 0330 SW Curry Street, Portland, OR 97201; 503-295-6422

ACS—Pennsylvania: (2 locations)

(Commonwealth Division, Inc.) Route 422 and Sipe Avenue, Hershey, PA 17033-0897; 717-533-6144

(Commonwealth Division, Inc.) 1626 Locust Street, Philadelphia, PA 19103; 215-985-5400

ACS—Puerto Rico (Puerto Rico Division, Inc.): Calle Alverio #577 Esquina Sargento Medina, Hato Rey, PR 00918; 787-764-2295

ACS—Rhode Island (Rhode Island Division, Inc.): 400 Main Street, Pawtucket, RI 02860; 401-722-8480

ACS—South Carolina (South Carolina Division, Inc.): 128 Stonemark Lane, Columbia, SC 29210-3855; 803-750-1693

ACS—South Dakota (South Dakota Division, Inc.): 4101 W. Carnegie Place, Sioux Falls, SD 57106-2322; 605-361-8277

ACS—Tennessee (Mid-South Division, Inc.): 1315 Eight Avenue South, Nashville, TN 37203; 615-255-1227

ACS—Texas (Texas Division, Inc.): 2433 Ridgepoint Drive, Austin, TX 78754; 512-928-2262

ACS—Utah (Utah Division, Inc.): 941 East 3300 South, Salt Lake City, UT 84106; 801-483-1500

ACS—Vermont (Vermont Division, Inc.): 13 Loomis Street, Montpelier, VT 05602; 802-223-2348

ACS—Virginia (Mid-Atlantic Division, Inc.): 4240 Park Place Court, Glen Allen, VA 23060; 804-527-3700

ACS—Washington (Western Pacific Division, Inc.): 2120 First Avenue North, Seattle, WA 98109-1140; 206-283-1152

ACS—West Virginia (Mid-Atlantic Division, Inc.): 2428 Kanawah Boulevard East, Charleston, WV 25311; 304-344-3611

ACS—Wisconsin (Wisconsin Division, Inc.): N19 W24350 Riverwood Drive, Waukesha, WI 53188; 414-523-5500

ACS—Wyoming (Wyoming Division, Inc.): 4202 Ridge Road, Cheyenne, WY 82001; 307-638-3331

Gilda Radner Familial Ovarian Cancer Registry
(800) OVARIAN or (716) 845-3110
Department of Gynecologic Oncology
Roswell Park Cancer Institute
Elm and Carlton Streets
Buffalo, NY 14263

Hereditary Cancer Institute
(402) 280-2942
Henry Lynch, MD
Creighton University School of Medicine
California at 24th
Omaha, Nebraska 68178

National Alliance of Breast Cancer Organizations
212-719-0154
1180 Avenue of the Americas
New York, New York 10036

National Cancer Institute
Cancer Information Service (CIS)
(800) 4-CANCER (9:00 AM–4:30 PM Monday through Friday)
Office of Cancer Communications
National Cancer Institute
Bethesda, MD 20892-2580

National Coalition for Cancer Survivorship
(301) 650-8868
1010 Wayne Avenue
Silver Spring, Maryland 20910

National Ovarian Cancer Coalition
561-393-3220
Gail Haywood, Executive Director
PO Box 4472
Boca Raton, Florida 33429

Oncology Nursing Society
412-921-7373
501 Holiday Drive
Pittsburgh, PA 15220-2749

National Cancer Institute-Designated Comprehensive and Clinical Cancer Centers

Alabama
University of Alabama at Birmingham
Comprehensive Cancer Center
(205) 934-5077
Wallace Tumor Institute, Room 235
1824 6th Avenue South
Birmingham, AL 35293-3300

Arizona
Arizona Cancer Center
(520) 626-2900
University of Arizona College of Medicine
1515 North Campbell Avenue
PO Box 245024
Tucson, AZ 85724-5024

California
City of Hope National Medical Center
(800) 826-HOPE (4673)
Beckman Research Institute
1500 East Duarte Road
Duarte, CA 91010

Irvine Clinical Cancer Center
(714) 456-8200
University of California at Irvine
Building 23, Route 81
101 The City Drive
Orange, CA 92668

Jonsson Comprehensive Cancer Center
(800) 825-2631
University of California at Los Angeles
1092 Wilshire Boulevard, Suite 1010
Los Angeles, CA 90024-6502

University of California at San Diego Cancer Center
(619) 543-3456
200 West Arbor Drive
San Diego, CA 92103-8421

USC/Norris Comprehensive Cancer Center
(800) 522-6237 or (213) 764-3000
University of Southern California
1441 Eastlake Avenue
Los Angeles, CA 90033-0800

Colorado
University of Colorado Cancer Center
(800) 473-2288
Campus Box B188
4200 East 9th Avenue
Denver. CO 80262

Connecticut
Yale Cancer Center
(203) 785-4095
Yale University School of Medicine
333 Cedar Street, Box 208028
New Haven, CT 06520-8028

District of Columbia
Lombardi Cancer Research Center
(202) 784-4000
Georgetown University Medical Center
3800 Reservoir Road, NW
Washington, DC 20007

Hawaii
Cancer Research Center of Hawaii
(808) 586-3013
University of Hawaii at Manoa
1236 Lauhala Street
Honolulu, HI 96813

Illinois
Robert H. Lurie Cancer Center
(312) 908-5250
Northwestern University
303 East Chicago Avenue
Chicago, IL 60611

University of Chicago Cancer Research Center
(312) 702-9200 or (800) 289-6333
5841 South Maryland Avenue
Chicago, IL 60637-1470

Maryland
The Johns Hopkins Oncology Center
(410) 955-8964
601 North Wolfe Street
Baltimore MD 21287

Massachusetts
Dana-Farber Cancer Institute
(617) 632-3476
44 Binney Street
Boston, MA 02115

Michigan
Barbara Ann Karmanos Cancer Institute
(313) 745-4400
110 East Warren Avenue
Detroit, MI 48201-1379

University of Michigan Comprehensive Cancer Center
(313) 936-9583 or (800) 865-1125
101 Simpson Drive
Ann Arbor, MI 48109-0752

Minnesota
Mayo Cancer Center
(507) 284-9589
200 1st Street SW
Rochester, MN 55905

Nebraska

Creighton University Hereditary Cancer Center
(402) 280-2941
2500 California Plaza
Omaha, NE 68178

New Hampshire
Norris Cotton Cancer Center
(603) 650-5527
Dartmouth-Hitchcock Medical Center
One Medical Center Drive, Hinman Box 7920
Lebanon, NH 03756-0001

New York

Albert Einstein College of Medicine
(718) 920-4826
Montefiore Medical Center
Department of Oncology
111 East 210th Street
Bronx, NY 10467

Herbert Irving Comprehensive Cancer Center
(212) 305-8610
6th Floor, Room 435
Milstein Hospital Building
177 Fort Washington Avenue
New York, NY 10032

Kaplan Comprehensive Cancer Center
(212) 263-6485
New York University Medical Center
550 1st Avenue
New York, NY 10016

Memorial Sloan-Kettering Cancer Center
(800) 525-2225
1275 York Avenue
New York, NY 10021

Roswell Park Cancer Institute
(800) ROSWELL (767-9355)
Elm and Carlton Streets
Buffalo, NY 14263-0001

University of Rochester Cancer Center
(716) 275-4911 or (800) 462-6763
Box 704
601 Elmwood Avenue
Rochester, NY 14642

North Carolina

Comprehensive Cancer Center of Wake Forest University
(910) 716-2255
Bowman Gray School of Medicine
Medical Center Boulevard
Winston-Salem, NC 27157-1082

Duke Comprehensive Cancer Center
(919) 684-3377
Duke University Medical Center
Box 3814
Durham, NC 27710

UNC Lineberger Comprehensive Cancer Center
(919) 966-3036 or (919) 966-1101
University of North Carolina School of Medicine
Campus Box 7295
102 West Drive
Chapel Hill, NC 27599-7295

Ohio
Case Western Reserve University/Ireland Cancer Center
(216) 844-5432 or (800) 641-2422
1110 Euclid Avenue
Cleveland, OH 44106-5065

Ohio State University Comprehensive Cancer Center
(614) 293-5066 or (800) 293-5066
Arthur G. James Cancer Hospital
and Research Institute
300 West Tenth Avenue
Columbus OH 43210-1240

Pennsylvania
Fox Chase Cancer Center
(215) 728-2570
7701 Burholme Boulevard
Philadelphia PA 19111

Kimmell Cancer Center
(800) 4-CNETWORK or 426-3895
Thomas Jefferson University
College Building, Suite 1014
1025 Walnut Street
Philadelphia, PA 19107

University of Pennsylvania Medical Center
(800) 383-UPCC or (215) 662-6364
6th Floor, Penn Tower
3400 Spruce Street
Philadelphia, PA 19104-4283

University of Pittsburgh Cancer Institute
(800) 237-4PCI (237-4724)
Information and Referral Service
Iroquois Building, Suite 405
3600 Forbes Avenue
Pittsburgh, PA 15213-2592

Tennessee
Drew-Meharry-Morehouse Consortium Cancer Center
(615) 327-6927
Meharry Medical College
1005 D.B. Todd Boulevard
Nashville, TN 37208

St. Jude Childrens Reserach Hospital
(901) 495-3300
332 North Lauderdale Street
Memphis, TN 38105-0318

Vanderbilt Cancer Center
(800) 811-8480 or (615) 936-1782
Vanderbilt University
649 Medical Research Building II
Nashville, TN 37232-6838

Texas
San Antonio Cancer Institute
(210) 616-5590
8122 Datapoint Drive, Suite 1000
San Antonio, TX 78229

The University of Texas
M.D. Anderson Cancer Center
(800) 392-1611
1515 Holcombe Boulevard
Houston, TX 77030

Utah
Huntsman Cancer Institute
(800) 488-2422
University of Utah
50 North Medical Drive
Salt Lake City, UT 84132

Vermont
Vermont Regional Cancer Center
(802) 656-4580
(802) 656-4414
University of Vermont
1 South Prospect Street
Burlington, VT 05401-3498

Virginia
Cancer Center at University of Virginia
(800) 223-9173 or (804) 924-2562
PO Box 334
Charlottesville, VA 22908

Massey Cancer Center
(804) 828-5116
Medical College of Virginia
Virginia Commonwealth University
Box 980037
401 College Street
Richmond, VA 23298-0037

Washington
Fred Hutchinson Cancer Research Center
(800) 804-8824
(206) 667-5000
Bone Marrow and Stem Cell Transplantation Information
1124 Columbia Street
Seattle, WA 98104

Wisconsin
University of Wisconsin Comprehensive Cancer Center
(608) 263-8090
600 Highland Avenue
Madison, WI 53792-0001

APPENDIX 3

Glossary of Terms

Acquired susceptibility mutation A mutation in a gene that occurs after birth from a carcinogenic insult.

Adenine A purine base found in RNA and DNA; one of the four chemical building blocks of RNA and DNA.

Allele One of several mutational forms of a specific gene. Most genes have two alleles, one on each copy of the chromosome.

Allozygote A diploid organism that has two genes at a particular locus which are not identical by descent from a common ancestor.

Amino acid Any one of a class of 20 molecules that combine to form proteins in living things.

Amniocentesis A procedure in which fluid is drawn from the amniotic sac in order to determine chromosomal abnormalities and the diagnosis of disease in the fetus.

Aneuploid A cell or organism possessing a chromosome number that is either more or less than the normal diploid amount. Aneuploid also describes cases in which the part of a chromosome is duplicated or deficient.

Anticodon Three nucleotides in transfer RNA that are complementary to the three bases of a specific codon in messenger RNA.

Asynapsis The partial or total failure of homologous chromosomes to pair during meiosis.

Atavism The reappearance of a trait possessed by a remote ancestor due to recessive genes or other masking characteristics.

ATP (adenosine triphosphate) A nucleotide that is involved in energy metabolism, is needed for RNA synthesis, occurs in all cells, and is used to store energy within a cell. It is composed of adenine, ribose, and phosphoric acid.

Autogamy Self-fertilization within the cell itself, resulting in homozygosity.

Autopolyploid A polyploid with more than two identical (or nearly identical) sets of chromosomes.

Autosomal dominant inheritance Inheritance of a gene, which is located on a chromosome other than the sex (X or Y) chromosome, and which in single state, may give rise to a phenotype that may be expressed through two or more generations.

Autosome Any chromosome except for the sex chromosomes "X" and "Y;" a chromosome not involved in sex determination.

Autozygote A diploid individual in which two genes of a locus are identical by descent from a common ancestral gene.

Base pair Two nitrogenous bases (consisting of either adenine and thymine or guanine and cytosine) that are held together by weak bonds. The bonds between base pairs hold the two strands of DNA together in the form of a double helix.

BRCA1 and BRCA2 The principal genes that indicate an inherited susceptibility to breast and ovarian cancers. These genes account for approximately 80% to 90% of all hereditary cases of breast cancer and the majority of hereditary ovarian cancer.

Carrier Someone with both a recessive, mutated gene (which is not expressed) and a normal copy of the gene. Carriers rarely develop diseases, but can pass the mutated gene on to their offspring.

Centromere Special region of a chromosome where spindle fiber attachment occurs during cell division.

Chromatid One of the two identical strands resulting from self-duplication of a chromosome during mitosis or meiosis.

Chromatin Made up of deoxyribonucleohistone (deoxyribonucleic acid connected to a protein structure base), chromatin is the carrier of genes in inheritance. This part of the cell nucleus stains easily.

Chromatography A method of separating chemical substances from each other and identifying the components from mixtures of molecules having similar properties.

Chromosome aberration Any abnormalities in either the structure or number of chromosomes. This includes deficiency, duplication, inversion, translocation, aneuploidy, polyploidy, as well as any other deviation from the norm.

Chromosome banding Staining chromosomes so that light and dark areas occur along the length of the chromosomes. Side by side comparisons identify pairs. Each chromosome can be identified by its banding pattern.

Chromosomes Structures located in the nucleus of a cell, which contain the genes. In a normal human being, chromosomes are paired; each cell has 46 chromosomes consisting of 22 pairs of autosomes and 2 sex chromosomes.

Clone The offspring of a single cell or organism derived by asexual reproduction.

Codominant alleles Alleles that are both completely expressed in the heterozygote.

Codon A set of three adjacent bases in a single strand of DNA or RNA.

Crossing over During meiosis, the breaking off of one maternal and one paternal chromosome, an exchange of corresponding segments of DNA, and the reunification of the chromosomes. This process can also result in a trade of alleles between chromosomes.

Cytogenetics Area of biology concerned with chromosomes and their implications for inherited characteristics.

Cytokinesis Changes that take place in the cytoplasm during cell division and other changes exclusive of nuclear division that are a part of mitosis or meiosis.

Cytoplasm The protoplasm of a cell outside the nucleus in which cell organelles (mitochondria, plastids, etc.) reside. It is the site of most of the chemical activities of the cell.

Cytosine A pyrimidine base found in RNA and DNA; also one of the four chemical building blocks of RNA and DNA.

Deficiency A lack or defect. Occurs when a segment of the chromosome is missing, reducing the number of loci.

Degeneracy Presence of more than one codon in the genetic code

Deletion loss or removal of a sequence of DNA with the regions on either side being joined together.

Diakinesis The stage of meiosis in which the bivalents become short and thick just before metaphase.

Dicentric chromosome A structurally abnormal chromosome having two centromeres.

Dimorphism The property of a group having two different forms as determined by characteristics such as sex, size or coloration.

Diploid A cell or organism having two sets of chromosomes.

Discordant Members of a pair showing different, instead of similar, characteristics.

DNA (deoxyribonucleic acid) A large molecule that carries the genetic information that cells need to replicate and to produce proteins; the substance of heredity. DNA is a polymer of nucleotides containing the sugar deoxyribose.

DNA sequence Determines the exact order of the base pairs in a segment of DNA.

Dominance Takes place when one member of an allele pair manifests itself to the exclusion of the other.

Endomitosis Occurs when the nucleus of a cell does not divide but the chromosomes duplicate themselves. This results in an increased chromosome number within the cell.

Enzyme A protein molecule that accelerates chemical reactions in cells or organisms.

Eukaryote A member of a large group of organisms whose cells have a true nucleus (nuclei enclosed by a membrane) and other well-developed subcellular components. The cells of all organisms except bacteria, blue-green algae and viruses are eukaryotic.

Euploid An individual or cell having a chromosome number that is the exact multiple of the haploid number. Having the proper amount of chromosomes for the cells of a particular species.

Exon A protein-coding sequence in a gene.

Expressivity The extent to which an inherited trait from a gene appears in an individual. The degree of expressivity varies in the individuals who carry the gene.

Familial adenomatous polyposis (FAP) An autosomal dominantly inherited predisposition to multiple adenomatous polyps of the colon and a risk for colorectal cancer that approaches 100% by age 60. The germ-line mutation for this disease is the APC gene, which stands for adenomatous polyposis coli. Other cancers, including papillary thyroid carcinoma, periampullary carcinoma, gastric cancer (particularly in FAP patients in Japan), small bowel cancer, pancreatic cancer, sarcomas and brain tumors, as well as desmoid tumors (which are not cancer) complicate this disease.

Fetus The unborn offspring of any viviparous animal in the postembryonic period until birth.

Frameshift Deletions or insertions that alter the three-base-pair frame in DNA that are translated into protein.

Gamete A male (sperm) or female (egg) reproductive cell.

Gene Segment of the DNA molecule and the fundamental biological unit of heredity. Genes contain chemical information to make proteins, control inherited bodily traits, or influence the activity of other genes.

Gene markers Landmarks for a target gene, either detectable traits that are inherited along with the gene or distinctive segments of DNA.

Gene mapping Determining the relative positions of genes on a chromosome and the distance between them.

Genetic linkage maps DNA maps that assign relative chromosomal locations to genetic landmarks—either genes for known traits or distinctive sequences of DNA—on the basis of how frequently they are inherited together.

Genome All the genetic material in an organism's chromosomes, which are inherited as a unit from one parent. All of the genetic information carried by a cell.

Genotype The entire genetic makeup of an organism.

Germ-line Cells having only a single set of chromosomes; specifically sperm and egg cells.

Germline mutation An alteration in the genetic material of the body's reproductive cells (egg or sperm) that becomes incorporated in the DNA of every cell in the body.

Glucocorticoid A steroid hormone that regulates gene expression in higher animals.

Guanine A purine base found in DNA and RNA; one of the four chemical building blocks of RNA and DNA.

Haploid An organism or cell having a single set of chromosomes or a genome.

Haplotype The specific combination of alleles in a defined region of a chromosome.

Hemizygous Having only one instead of a pair of genes of a particular kind due to a loss of DNA. This condition is normal in sex linkage.

Hereditary nonpolyposis colorectal cancer (HNPCC) Autosomal dominantly inherited disease predisposing to colorectal cancer on a site-specific basis (Lynch syndrome I) and in association with a variety of extracolonic cancers (carcinoma of the endometrium, ovary, stomach, small bowel, and pancreas, and transitional-cell carcinoma) of the ureter and renal pelvis (Lynch syndrome II). Genes identified in this syndrome include hMSH2, hMLH1, hPMS1, and hPMS2.

Heredity Transmission of traits from parents to offspring. The genetic constitution of an individual.

Heritability Degree to which a given trait is controlled by inheritance

Heteroploid An individual with an abnormal number (anything other than the haploid or diploid amount) of chromosomes.

Heterozygote An organism with different alleles at one or more loci on homologous chromosomes.

Histone A simple protein containing many basic groups occurring in the nucleus of most higher organisms.

"Holandric" gene Transmitted only by genes located on the Y chromosome. Inherited exclusively through male descent.

Homologous chromosomes Chromosomes acquired from the male and female parent that come in pairs of similar in shape and size.

Homozygosity The state of possessing a pair of identical alleles at a given locus.

Homozygous A patient with identical alleles at the same locus of homologous chromosomes is said to be homozygous.

Human genome The complete set of genes necessary to produce a human being.

Hybrid An organism produced from homozygous parents differing in one or more genes.

Hybridization Interbreeding of species, races, varieties among plants or animals; a process of forming a hybrid by cross pollination of plants or by mating animals of different types. Also known as crossbreeding.

Incomplete dominance Takes place when both members of an allele pair manifest themselves. The heterozygote can be distinguished by either of its homozygous parents.

Incomplete penetrance Absence of expression of the phenotype in an obligate gene carrier.

Inherited susceptibility mutation A mutation in a gene that is inherited in Mendelian fashion, and thus present in all cells in the body from birth, which causes susceptibility to a given disease.

Insertion The gain or addition of a sequence(s) of DNA not normally present.

Interphase The interval between two successive cell divisions, the period in a cell cycle when DNA is replicated in the nucleus; it is followed by mitosis.

Intron A noncoding intervening sequence in a gene. The sequences are transcribed into RNA, but are eliminated from the message before it is translated into protein.

Inversion A rearrangement that reverses the order of a linear array of genes on a chromosome.

Karyotype The chromosome characteristics of an individual or cell line. Chromosomes arranged in order of length and according to position of centromere. Important in the diagnosis of certain hereditary diseases.

Kindred Individuals who are related by genetics or marriage to all other members of the particular group ("kindred is often used interchangeably with "family").

Lethal allele An allele that causes the cell or organism that possesses it to become incapable of survival.

Linkage The proximity of two or more genes on a chromosome; the closer together the genes are, the less likely it becomes that they will be separated during DNA repair or replication processes, and the more likely it becomes that they will be inherited together.

Linkage analysis Genes are said to be "linked" when they reside close together on the same chromosome. Statistical analysis of linkage of two genes is then expressed as a Lod score.

Linkage map A diagram that shows the relative positions (loci) of genes on a chromosome as determined by genetic analysis.

Locus (plural loci) The position of a gene or allele on a chromosome.

Meiosis A special method of cell division by which the chromosome number of a sex cell becomes reduced to half the diploid number of somatic cells. This results in the formation of gametes and is a vital source of variability through recombination.

Mesoderm The middle layer of three primary germ layers that forms in the early animal embryo and gives rise to such parts including bone, blood, blood vessels and connective tissue among others.

Messenger RNA (mRNA) Serves as a template and carries information necessary for protein synthesis from DNA.

Metabolic cell A cell that is not dividing.

Metacentric chromosome Having the centromere in the middle so that the arms are approximately equal in length.

Metaphase A stage in mitosis or meiosis during which the chromosomes are aligned along the equatorial plane of the cell and the dividing chromosomes can be made visible.

Mitochondria Spherical to rod shaped organelles found in the cytoplasm of cells. They are the principal sites where oxidative phosphorylation takes place to produce ATP.

Mitosis The severing of duplicated chromosomes and division of the cytoplasm produces daughter cells that are genetically identical to each other and to the parent cell.

Monohybrid The offspring of two homozygous parents that differ from one another in that each is homozygous for a different allele at only one gene locus.

Monozygotic twins Identical twins (born from the same egg).

Multiple alleles A condition in which a particular gene occurs in three or more allelic forms in a population of organisms.

Mutable genes Genes which have an abnormally high mutation rate.

Mutagen A chemical or physical agent that is capable of inducing genetic mutations by causing changes in DNA. Most mutagens are carcinogens.

Mutant A gene or organism that has undergone a permanent alteration in genetic structure.

Mutation Any permanent variation in genetic material when occurring in germ cells. This heritable change will be passed from parent to offspring. If the mutation occurs in somatic cells, it is not transmitted to the offspring.

Nonsense mutation Any change in DNA that results in a three-base-pair sequence that does not code for an amino acid and thus terminates the protein sequence.

Nucleic acid A large molecule composed of phosphoric acid, pentose sugar, and organic bases. Either RNA or DNA. Exerts primary control over life processes in all organisms.

Nucleotide The basic unit of DNA and RNA, consisting of a phosphate, a ribose sugar and a purine or pyrimidine base in an exact order.

Nucleus The genetic material (chromosomes) contained within the cellular organelle and the component that regulates cellular activity in eukaryotes.

Null Mutation A mutation that abolishes the expression of a gene.

Oncogenes Genes that, when mutated, can advance the growth of cancer and are thus associated with cancer. When normal, these genes play a role in the regulating the growth of cells.

Palliative An alleviating treatment that can give relief, but is not a cure.

Pedigree A family history in diagram form showing the family members (males as squares, females as circles) and their relationships to affected individuals; those affected by a particular illness are denoted by "filled-in" symbols.

Penetrance The extent to which the inheritance of a mutated gene results in illness or other physiologic manifestation. The proportion of individuals with the genotype (such as hMSH2 germ-line carriers of HNPCC) who manifest the phenotype. A gene is considered to be completely penetrant if it is always associated with illness, and incompletely penetrant if it is not.

Peptides Form the constituent parts of proteins. They contain amino acids and are a breakdown or buildup unit in protein metabolism.

Phenotype The observable physical or biochemical characteristics of an organism, as determined by both genetic makeup and environmental influences.

Plasma membrane The membrane surrounding a cell.

Polymer Compound that results from a chemical union of two or more molecules of the same kind, and has the same elements in the same proportions but with a higher molecular weight and different physical properties.

Polymerase An enzyme that catalyzes the formation of nucleic acids. It is involved in the synthesis of large molecules within the cell for the transfer of genetic information.

Polymorphism Two or more kinds of physiological individuals maintained in a breeding population.

Polynucleotide A linear series of connected nucleotides occurring in DNA or RNA.

Polypeptide A linear molecule having two or more amino acids and at least one peptide group. Such molecules are referred to as dipeptides, tripeptides, tetrapeptides, etc., depending on the number of amino acids present.

Polyploid Any organism, individual, or cell having more than two full sets of homologous chromosomes. There might be three (triploid), four (tetraploid), five (pentaploid), six (hexaploid), seven (heptaploid), or eight (octoploid).

Predicative gene tests Gene testing to identify abnormalities that may cause a person to be vulnerable to certain diseases or disorders.

Prokaryote A member of a large group of organisms (including bacteria and blue-green algae) that lack a true nucleus, nuclear membrane, and cannot undergo meiosis. Instead, they reproduce by cell fission —cells split into two identical daughter cells and become a new, independent organism.

Promoter mutation Any mutation in that part of DNA involved in binding of RNA polymerase to initiate transcription.

Prophase During mitosis, the stage at which the chromosomes become visible since the chromosome is longitudinally double except in the region of the centromere, the cell nucleus starts to lose its identity, and the centrioles divide and begin to migrate.

Protein A large, complex molecule made of amino acid chains. Each protein has a unique, genetically defined amino acid sequence which determines its specific shape and function. Proteins (such as antibodies, hormones and enzymes) are necessary for the regulation, structure, and function of the body.

Proto-oncogene A normal cellular gene that with alteration, such as by mutation or DNA rearrangement, can become an active oncogene.

Recessive One member of an allelic pair incapable of expression when the other (dominant) allele is present. Only if the responsible allele is carried by both members of a pair of homologous chromosomes can the recessive allele manifest itself.

Recombination The formation of new combinations of genes not found in the parents due to crossing over between homologous chromosomes during meiosis.

Regulator gene A gene that dictates the expression of another gene or genes.

Remission Both the decrease and apparent disappearance of disease, and the period during which this occurs.

Replication Duplicating an exact copy of a strand of RNA or DNA.

Ribosomes Organelles in the cytoplasm on which proteins are synthesized by the cell.

RING finger motif Zinc finger motif, a structure seen in many DNA-binding proteins, composed of a loop of polypeptide chain held in a hairpin bend bound to a zinc atom.

RNA (ribonucleic acid) Similar to DNA in structure. The many types of RNA serve important roles in protein synthesis. RNA is a nucleic acid containing the sugar ribose.

Sensitivity Analytical: The probability that a test will detect an analyte when it is present in a specimen. Clinical: The probability that a person with a disease, or who will develop a disease, will have a positive test result.

Somatic cell Includes any cells of the body, with the exception of germline cells.

Specificity Analytical: The probability that a test will be negative when an analyte is absent from a specimen. Clinical: The probability that a test will be negative in person free of a disease, and who will not develop the disease.

Splice mutation A mutation resulting from imprecise removal of introns and joining of exons in RNA.

Stem cell A mitotically active somatic cell from which other cells arise by differentiation.

Stop codon A three-base-pair sequence in DNA that does not code for an amino acid, and thus results in termination of the protein sequence.

Thymine A pyrimidine base found only in DNA; also one of the four chemical building blocks of DNA.

Transcription Synthesis of RNA on a DNA template.

Transgenic Term applied to organisms that have been altered by introducing DNA molecules into them from other organisms.

Translation Synthesis of a protein on an RNA template.

Translocation The repositioning of a segment of a chromosome from its usual site to another in the genome (either on the same chromosome or another one).

Tumor-suppressor genes Normally, these genes restrict cell growth, but when missing or inactivated by mutation, they permit cells to grow without restraint.

Uracil A pyrimidine base found only in RNA; one of the four chemical building blocks of RNA.

Variable expressivity Difference in the phenotype, such as the age or onset of specific type of cancer, in an obligate germ-line carrier.

Wild-type allele Normal allele of a gene, which has not undergone any mutation.

Index